Endorsements for
***Reducing the Risk of Alzheimer's***

"Dr. Savage's program is currently the best strategy for reducing the risk of this dreaded disease."

—Robert F. Cathcart III, MD

"A book that accurately documents complementary approaches to premature senility is much needed and overdue. Michael Savage's book is a most valuable contribution."

—Russel Jaffe, MD, PhD, Fellow,
Health Studies Collegium

"Dr. Savage's book does the best job yet of showing the potential dangers of aluminum. Now we find it is yet another pollutant that may be doing us in. Its correction is a matter of choice—your choice. Dr. Savage gives you the facts to help make that choice rational and effective."

—Richard Kunin, MD

"I recommend that everyone not following these nutritional (orthomolecular) principles—especially if there is a family history—should read this book and take its message very seriously."

—A. Hoffer, MD, PhD

# REDUCING *the* RISK *of* ALZHEIMER'S

## ALUMINUM AND THE BRAIN

# REDUCING *the* RISK *of* ALZHEIMER'S

## ALUMINUM AND THE BRAIN

**MICHAEL SAVAGE**
MS, MA, PhD

Post Hill
PRESS

A POST HILL PRESS BOOK
ISBN: 979-8-89565-650-1
ISBN (eBook): 979-8-89565-651-8

Reducing the Risk of Alzheimer's:
Aluminum and the Brain


Cover design by Conroy Accord

This book contains advice and information relating to health care. It should be used to supplement rather than replace the advice of your doctor or another trained health professional. You are advised to consult your health professional with regard to matters related to your health, and in particular regarding matters that may require diagnosis or medical attention. The purpose of this book is to provide an interesting overview to the general public concerning Alzheimer's Disease, as it appears in the scientific literature. All efforts have been made to assure the accuracy of the information in this book as of the date of publication. The publisher and the author disclaim liability for any medical outcomes that may occur as a result of applying the methods suggested in this book.



Post Hill Press

Post Hill Press
New York • Nashville
posthillpress.com

Published in the United States of America
1 2 3 4 5 6 7 8 9 10

# Contents

## PART 2: Solutions

# List of Tables

# INTRODUCTION

*New Introduction:* Reducing the Risk of Alzheimer's *by Michael Savage, Ph.D.*

This book was first published in 1987 in hardcover by Stein and Day. At the time, it was forty years ahead of its time. It was reprinted in 1989, and later in a private edition in 2007.

That's just the background.

When this book first came out, it was considered "out there" because, for the first time in a popular format, I presented the connection between aluminum and other metals with Alzheimer's disease. Even then, scientific progress in this area was advancing rapidly. Of course, the medical establishment scoffed and ignored it.

At the time, I was the director of the Alzheimer's Research Institute and conducting an epidemiological study on the disease. Alzheimer's was then the fourth leading cause of death in the United States. It remains one of the most feared diseases, because when you lose your memory and no longer recognize your loved ones, you essentially lose your soul.

Recent research has not only supported my original hypothesis about the dangers of neurotoxic aluminum, but progress in this field is now moving rapidly.

German researchers have shown that, although exposure to dangerous aluminum compounds in foods has been decreasing, we still ingest more aluminum than experts consider safe. This book is about minimizing exposure to aluminum compounds. Aluminum is present in many products, including food, cosmetics, baking tools, and, of course, aluminum foil.

Aluminum compounds are also found in drinking water (where they are used to purify it) and in processed foods, where they serve various purposes such as emulsifiers and colorants. Strangely enough, even fresh fruits and vegetables sometimes contain aluminum due to soil contamination from human activities such as mining. Deodorants often contain aluminum salts, and the metal is present in baking trays and other cooking utensils.

The fact remains: aluminum is neurotoxic, and we need to reduce our intake of it. While this book primarily focuses on eliminating aluminum from our lives, it goes far beyond that. It was the first popular book to address nutrition for a healthy brain. Beyond aluminum, I discuss missing nutrients that can reduce risk—vitamins, minerals, amino acids, and fish oils, which are now considered essential in preventing Alzheimer's disease.

One of the most interesting new studies comes from researchers at the University of Southern California, who discovered potential new drug targets for Alzheimer's disease. They found that a shortage of HDL "good" cholesterol in the brain increases the risk of Alzheimer's. This shortage is linked to dysfunction in ABCA1, a protein responsible for producing HDL when working properly.

In Alzheimer's patients, ABCA1 was found to be trapped inside a part of the cell responsible for clearing waste. This malfunction was associated with a rise in a harmful form of cholesterol known as oxysterol. Lowering oxysterol levels in both animal models and human stem cells freed the trapped ABCA1 and restored normal cellular function. The researchers propose that lowering oxysterol may be a promising new way to prevent or treat Alzheimer's disease.

Their findings also suggest that early changes in Alzheimer's disease may begin long before the hallmark buildup of amyloid plaques and tau tangles. As Dr. Yassine explained, "if we ask why amyloid and tau accumulate, a plausible explanation is that the brain's waste recycling system is failing. Drugs that lower oxysterols may help prevent the disease from advancing."

This research highlights new frontiers, including early detection through blood tests, voice analysis, and remote EEG monitoring. The immune system also appears to play an important role, and genetic factors—including rare protective mutations—are being studied as well.

But the key question is: what are the prevention strategies? That is what my book is all about. The latest research identifies lifestyle and other modifiable risk factors for Alzheimer's, such as diet, exercise, and cognitive training.

This book covers them all. We also now know that aluminum may compete with lithium in certain biological processes. Lithium, long used to treat bipolar disorder, is now being studied as a preventive for Alzheimer's. Unlike aluminum, which is purely toxic, lithium has neuroprotective effects at trace levels and may even promote neurogenesis. Some studies suggest that lithium reduces the DNA damage inflicted by aluminum.

To summarize: aluminum has no beneficial role in the human body and is potentially toxic, while lithium may help protect the brain from aluminum's harmful effects.

In addition to metals, you should know that several common over-the-counter and prescription medications may increase dementia risk. These include:

Antihistamines like Benadryl, which block acetylcholine—a neurotransmitter vital for learning and memory.

Opioids, including those used in anesthesia, which can nearly double dementia risk within years of surgery.

Proton pump inhibitors like omeprazole (Prilosec), which may affect vitamin B12 absorption and beta-amyloid buildup.

Benzodiazepines like Valium and Xanax, which depress brain function and impair memory when used long-term.

Tricyclic antidepressants, which have anticholinergic effects that may be linked to dementia risk.

Always consult your physician before stopping any medication, but be aware of these risks.

In conclusion, *Reducing the Risk of Alzheimer's* was decades ahead of its time in both prevention and mitigation of Alzheimer's disease and other dementias. While it focuses on aluminum as a neurotoxin, it also offers a groundbreaking chapter on nutrition for brain health—a chapter that remains as relevant today as ever.

When first published, this book was endorsed by leading researchers. Dr. Robert F. Cathcart II, MD, wrote: "Dr. Savage's program is currently the best strategy for reducing the risk of this dreaded disease."

Dr. Richard Kunin, MD, said: "This book does the best job yet of showing the potential dangers of aluminum... Dr. Savage gives you the facts to make your choices rational and effective."

Finally, Dr. Abram Hoffer, MD, PhD, called it "a very valuable contribution to the literature" and urged that everyone with a family history of Alzheimer's take its message seriously.

# PART 1

# The Problem

# 1

# THE ALZHEIMER'S PROBLEM

Alzheimer's disease is the sixth leading cause of death in the United States and affects people in considerable numbers all over the world, but it was not isolated from other bodily disabilities and given a name until 1906 when this terrible condition was first described by the German physician Alois Alzheimer.

The devastating collection of symptoms now called Alzheimer's disease did not get reported in the medical literature in centuries prior to this one. It can therefore be assumed that if it existed, it was extremely rare.

How does a "new" disease happen to become the sixth largest killer of people? What's new in this world that might be connected with the appearance and rapid spread of a non-contagious disease?

Recent studies have shown that in the autopsies of the brains of people who have died from Alzheimer's, there is a much higher concentration of aluminum than is normal. Alzheimer's is a twentieth-century phenomenon. And aluminum is a twentieth-century metal that a great many of us ingest unknowingly when we cook in aluminum pots and pans, use over-the-counter antacids and analgesics that are buffered with aluminum, wrap food in aluminum foil for later consumption, eat yogurt and other supposedly healthful foods kept fresh by aluminum foil, and drink quantities of soda and beer that have been swishing around in aluminum cans.

In any profession in which common sense predominated, the appearance of aluminum, which could not be efficiently refined before the late nineteenth century, and the catastrophic epidemic of Alzheimer's during the same period, would cause plain logic to suggest that the "coincidence" should be examined forthrightly and with the highest possible priority for scientific investigators.

However, medicine is one of the most conservative of professions. It is understandable that after doctors get out of medical school and complete their internships, their lives become occupied with heavy-duty practice and too little time to keep up with all of the literature on the explosive developments in medicine. For instance, the field of cancer research is progressing so rapidly that a significant number of patients who would not have stood a chance of remission or cure five years ago can today lead useful lives because of techniques developed in the last five years. How can a general practitioner or an internist or a specialist in any field except oncology (the cancer specialty) know all there is to know in such a rapidly advancing field?

The same, of course, is true of other fields. Most notably, nutrition. At best, doctors get just a few hours of training in nutrition, so what they know is understandably not much different from what their grandfathers knew about eating balanced meals. Yet today, scientific developments in the field of nutrition are saving lives, prolonging lives, keeping people out of mental institutions, and yet while laymen and specialists in nutrition were seizing these new findings and putting them to use in their own lives and in those of others, physicians, conservative as always, seemed to be in the rearguard instead of the vanguard of one of the most effective health revolutions in the history of man.

Conservative medicine is constantly playing catch-up. It has taken nearly thirty years for the cancer establishment to accept the link between diet and cancer, and only recently have we seen the American Cancer Society and the National Cancer Institute offer any dietary guidelines to reduce our risk of succumbing to this disease. My concern is with the millions whose lives might have been prolonged or saved not only by early detection but by earlier investigation and acceptance of the clues that have been around for a generation. It doesn't do the patient any good after he is dead to know that a slow-moving field will find incontrovertible evidence that a cure works. We need a faster response to operate faster vehicles, whether on land or in the air. We need a faster response to save lives now in the fast-moving field of medicine.

More than a decade ago good epidemiological studies clearly pointed to the link between diets too rich in saturated fats and coronary heart disease. These weren't secret studies conducted by amateurs. They were published studies conducted by professionals. Yet only in the past few years has the medical and biomedical research community begun to recommend the dietary practices necessary to lower the high incidence of heart disease among Americans and others who consume far too much saturated fats in their diets.

And so it has been with Alzheimer's. *The dietary links to Alzheimer's disease have appeared in print since the 1930s.* Now, half a century later, we are taking notice of the self-destructive practices by means of which we have been quite literally poisoning ourselves and assaulting the one human organ for which there is no transplant remedy—the brain.

The reluctance to accept new discoveries is not an American phenomenon, nor is it confined to medicine. In Britain, when Charles Darwin and Alfred Russel Wallace first presented their theory of evolution to the Royal Geographic Society in London, the reigning master of that scientific body cast his imperious eyes at the two young men and in his stentorian voice addressed them. "All that is old in what you say is true," he said, "and all that is new is false." That motivated young Darwin to present his ideas in a book aimed not at his fellow scientists but at the educated public. And so he published *On the Origin of the Species.*

If we take a close look at the history of medicine, we find that about half of the accepted truths of one generation are discarded in the next generation. If the gospels of medicine are only half true at any given time, it behooves the person concerned with his or her health to go for a better batting average than the medical community by keeping as informed as possible about new developments. And it behooves me to address not only my fellow professionals, some of whose minds are very open indeed, but the general public, whose need to know overrides all others: We're glad that posterity will advance in its knowledge, but right now we're out to prolong and improve our own lives, and we're all in favor of early-warning systems that make good sense.

This book proposes a *risk-reduction program* for one of the most widespread, devastating diseases ever to be inflicted upon mankind, Alzheimer's disease. It is a book for those who fear they may succumb to this disease; it is also a book for those with an ever-growing awareness of the correlation among our nutritional intake, our environment, and its effect on our bodies.

While much that is offered in this book is based upon good, theoretical evidence and logic, there is also some hard data available from clinical studies. These were undertaken by Dr. Richard Casdorph, M.D., Ph.D., an internist and cardiologist in Long Beach, California. I will report on the results of fifteen of Dr. Casdorph's patients who were suffering with various brain disorders, including Alzheimer's disease, and the excellent results and improvements he achieved using chelation to remove aluminum from the brains of sufferers of these diseases.

On a research trip to Japan I learned of the exciting work of Yoshiro Yase, M.D., Division of Neurological Diseases, Wakayama Medical College. This keen scientist has long held that aluminum may be a key player in the riddle of the disease ALS (amyotrophic lateral sclerosis) as it appears in the people of the Kii Peninsula of Japan and among certain groups on Guam. As you will read later in this book, these people contract ALS, which is similar in many key respects to Alzheimer's disease, the similarity being the physical and mental symptoms and the clinical findings of large quantities of aluminum deposited in that portion of the brain that controls the functions that are diminished in Alzheimer's disease. As I was fortunate to learn from Dr. Yase, the soil and water in Guam and the regions where ALS is found in Japan is highly dense with aluminum, and at the same time, local soils, drinking water, and foods are low in calcium and magnesium. These latter deficiencies, as we will show, tend to attract aluminum into brain cells.

Interesting from the point of view of a nutrition-oriented risk-reduction program for Alzheimer's disease is the discovery that with the introduction of foods rich in calcium and magnesium, over a twenty-year period, the disease ALS has largely disappeared in Guam! By learning how to reduce our intake of aluminum and other toxic metals, while correcting possible mineral imbalances, we will be establishing a prudent risk-reduction program for ourselves and others.

While the news about aluminum and the other minerals is being discussed and investigated in Japan and Canada, the official word in most conventional medical circles continues to be that aluminum is not at all implicated in Alzheimer's disease.

Ostriches see what they want to see, even if they have to bury their heads in the sand to avoid seeing some things.

In the April 10, 1986, issue of the *New England Journal of Medicine*, there is a review article titled "Medical Progress in Alzheimer's Disease," by Robert Katzman, M.D. While this article is an excellent depiction of the manifestations of the disease, there is, in fact, no medical progress reported. The following quote appears in the text, "There is no evidence that exposure to such sources of exogenous aluminum, as aluminum in antacids, antiperspirants, or even the large amount used in renal dialysis, increases the risk of Alzheimer's disease. Thus a direct relation between exogenous aluminum, and aluminum deposits in the brain of persons with Alzheimer's disease, has not been established." Note the use of the words "has not been established."

Neither has it been proven that exogenous aluminum is *un*related to the deposition of aluminum in the brains of persons with Alzheimer's disease! Numerous articles outlining the toxic effects of aluminum on brain tissue have existed in the literature for many, many, years.

In fact, several recently published articles directly suggest that we "should" reduce aluminum intake in patients with Alzheimer's disease. A notable article is by Armand Lione, Ph.D., of the Associated Pharmacologists and Toxicologists in Washington.

Another is an article by H. M. Wisniewski and coworkers of the Department of Pathological Neurobiology and Pathological Biochemistry of the New York State Institute for Basic Research in Developmental Disabilities, Staten Island, New York. In their article, the following is clearly stated, "Today, aluminum has been implicated in the following human disorders: 1) Pre-senile and senile dementia of the Alzheimer's type, 2) Amyotrophic Lateral Sclerosis (ALS) and Parkinsonism dementia (PD) Complex, 3) Dialysis dementia (DD), 4) Some forms of Epilepsy."

Dr. Wisniewski reports, in his article entitled "Aluminum and the Central Nervous System," that the interest in the toxic effects of aluminum began in the late 1890s when compounds derived from aluminum were first used in foods such as baking powder. We learned that the curiosity of neuroscientists was aroused regarding the effects of aluminum in 1942, when it was shown that by applying the metal to the cortex of monkeys, a "chronic state of convulsive activity with recurrent seizures, that simulated epilepsy in man" was produced.

Reading Dr. Wisniewski's article further, we learn that "Aluminum drew the attention of brain researchers for the second time in 1965 when Doctors Klatzo, Terry, and Wisniewski reported that aluminum salts induced so called neurofibrillary changes in rabbit nerve cells."

These are some of the many interesting cases and studies implicating aluminum in Alzheimer's disease that are completely ignored by Dr. Katzman. Others are: Dr. David Shore and coworkers, "Aluminum Flouride Complexes—Preclinical Studies"; Dr. George Trapp, "Aluminum Binding to Organic Acids and Plasma Proteins. Implications for Dialysis Encephalopathy"; Dr. Armand Lione, "The Reduction of Aluminum Intake in Patients With Alzheimer's Disease"; Dr. Herta Spencer and coworkers, "Effects of Aluminum Hydroxide on Flouride and Calcium Metabolism"; Dr. Gilbert H. Mayor and coworkers, "Aluminum Metabolism and Toxicity in Renal Failure; A Review."

All of the above articles are found in a single issue of an excellent scientific journal, the *Journal of Environmental Pathology, Toxicology & Oncology*, Volume 6, Number 1, Sept./Oct. 1985, under a banner headline entitled "Clinical Implications of Aluminum Neurotoxicity."

Not one of these excellent articles is mentioned in the Katzman review article in the *New England Journal of Medicine.*

Let's look at it another way. There have been many more scientific articles condemning cigarette smoking as a severe health risk than the recent articles on the hazards of aluminum. But with all the warnings we *now* hear, I can't help remembering that full-color ad that used to appear in national magazines with the headline, "More doctors smoke Camels than any other cigarette." The researchers whose work I referred to above have news that is vital to our health right now, and I have no intention of keeping the information in this book secret while the old-line establishmentarians and their uncreative colleagues in medical research stick to the comfort of their flat-earth theories.

At a time when too many conventional medical practitioners are unable or unwilling to offer clear preventive advice for this and other diseases, it is necessary that *the best evidence for cause and cure be examined and a rational risk-reduction program outlined.* I have set forth in this book a clear outline of both the disease and what the reader can do to reduce the risks.

The reader is advised to read the following pages and then discuss them with the family physician. For this purpose a key to the best scientific papers is presented in the bibliography.

But in the meantime, if what you read makes sense, get rid of your aluminum pots and pans, make sure you get the nutrients described in detail later in this book, and stop ingesting aluminum in over-the-counter medications, all of which have nonaluminum counterparts. All it takes is reading the labels before you buy. If you're one step ahead of the next fellow in reducing your risk, I'm all for it. And if your doctor, on reading the recommended scientific articles agrees, so much the better for him and his other patients.

This book offers concrete advice, not false hope. And one piece of that concrete advice is stay ahead of the ostriches who dispense false despair. Give yourself the best possible chance in life for resisting Alzheimer's and for knowing that there is a treatment available today that is worth trying for those who have already been condemned for a life without a working brain, a condition that is sometimes worse than death, and that debilitates not only the patient but his or her spouse and family who must care for a person who becomes an unperson before their very eyes.

2

# WHAT *IS* ALZHEIMER'S DISEASE?

The phone awoke Arlene and her husband in the early morning hours. It was Arlene's father, his voice filled with desperation. "Your mother is hysterical," he said. "I can't do anything with her....She says she doesn't love me anymore....Says this is her house and I have to get out....She tells me there's another woman in the house. Of course there's no other woman in the house. Would you talk to her, please? Try to calm her down?"

Things happened quickly after that—an ambulance trip to the nearest hospital, then a longer trip to a large city hospital where Jane, Arlene's mother, was locked behind doors in the psychiatric ward for two weeks. Finally the journey ended at a nursing home with Jane having been diagnosed as suffering from Alzheimer's disease. It is an organic form of senile dementia (the medical term for progressive mental deterioration), in which the brain cells degenerate causing a loss in mental function and turning vital, active, intelligent human beings into vacant, helpless shells. It is regarded generally as an insidious, slowly progressive condition, affecting both males and females equally. While symptomatically similar to senile dementia, the notable difference is the earlier age of onset.

Alzheimer's disease can occur in the prime of life, attacking people during their fifties or sixties. It is also the major cause of senility today. It is estimated that Alzheimer's disease affects between 5 percent and 15 percent of all Americans over the age of sixty-five, a total of 1.2 to 4 million people. As more people are living longer, the disease is progressing at an epidemic rate. After coronary heart disease, cancer, and strokes, it is the sixth leading cause of death in this country.

As the brain deteriorates in Alzheimer's disease, muscle spasms and convulsions may occur. Death may result from such seizures or, more commonly, from associated secondary conditions such as infections.

Alzheimer's disease exacts a tremendous toll in human and financial resources. Patients need constant care, supervision, and support. The emotional and financial costs to the victims' families are immeasurable. However, the disease is also draining our nation's financial resources. More than half of the 1.3 million Americans in nursing homes are Alzheimer's sufferers, their costs reaching some $13 billion a year.

## How Does Alzheimer's Disease Start? What Are Its Signs and Symptoms?

The patient Jane, mentioned previously, was only sixty-two when she first started showing evidence of Alzheimer's disease. She and her husband had recently retired from farming. They had worked hard, saved, and invested their money wisely. It was the time in their life when they could finally afford to fulfill their lifelong dreams. The children were grown and living successful lives; now they could afford to do anything THEY wished. But rather than reaping the rewards of their long, hard years of labor, they were plunged into the endless nightmare of the living death of Alzheimer's.

Alzheimer's disease begins insidiously and progresses slowly but inexorably, until the sufferer cannot attend to the simplest details of self-care and may not even remember his or her name. Although the symptoms may vary from patient to patient and from day to day in an individual, there are certain common features in all patients, and the disease follows a somewhat predictable path.

Initially, the victim may just exhibit a lack of energy, drive, and initiative, and neither he nor his family may be aware that anything is really wrong. The individual may just avoid new challenges and seek refuge in familiar situations. For example, he may want to visit only family members and close, old friends rather than go to new places and meet new people.

However, with time, greater changes in mental function and behavior begin to appear, and the disease can traditionally be divided into three clinical stages. The first obvious symptom or stage is forgetfulness. The individual will forget the names of persons well known to him; he will also be unable to remember where he puts various objects, such as the car keys or his wallet, or what day of the week, month, or year it is. He will start forgetting to attend appointments he has made or get lost trying to find places that were once very familiar. In the beginning, such episodes of forgetfulness may just be minor annoyances to the individual and his family, and he may still be able to function reasonably well. Eventually though, lapses of memory will become debilitating.

The patient Jane had once been a marvelous cook, but with the development of Alzheimer's disease she forgot how to cook and could not even remember how to turn on the stove. She would frequently get lost trying to find the supermarket, beauty shop, or the car, or different rooms in the house. She would forget which TV program she had watched or whether she had eaten anything recently. Another patient would forget to get off the bus at his stop or would get off and then walk in the wrong direction.

Memory loss at first affects mostly the short-term memory, but gradually, it affects the long-term memory as well. The patient must be continuously monitored, or he may wander off and become hopelessly lost. The patient's speech slows down, and he loses the thread of conversation or forgets which words he wanted to use. He may also lose other mental functions and learned skills such as the ability to do arithmetic calculations.

With time, the deterioration becomes more serious, and the victim enters the second stage in which, along with forgetfulness, he shows signs of confusion and disorientation and may develop changes in personality and irritability. He may ramble during conversation, repeating the same statements over and over, or make up words of his own. He may do unexpected things, like putting his clothes on backward or eating unsuitable foods such as flowers. He loses a sense of time and may be unable to sleep soundly, causing him to wander at nights. The patient gradually becomes unable to carry out routine chores or to make any decisions and plan ahead. Although his deterioration becomes progressively much more obvious, the sufferer loses recognition of or concern for his problems. He becomes insensitive to the feelings of other people.

Typically, after the early stages, the victim denies to himself and others the changes that are taking place. But anxiety may eventually override this denial in stressful situations, and the victim may become overtly nervous. He may also become depressed.

In the final third stage of the disease, the patient suffers total loss of intellectual ability and is completely unable to cope on his own. He cannot take care of himself, and everything must be done for him, such as bathing, shaving, cleaning his teeth, dressing, and feeding. He may not recognize the physical need to urinate or defecate and may need to be taken to the bathroom regularly. The patient may be restless and active but without any purpose. At other times he may sit silently and stare blankly for hours on end.

The Alzheimer's victim may be afflicted with delusions and become emotionally disturbed. He may develop paranoid traits and jealous rages as Jane did. The sufferer may become aggressive, hostile, and violent to those around him, despite all their efforts to care for the individual, and sorely try their patience.

The victim may also exhibit an increased interest in sexual activity (even after years of inactivity). He may masturbate frequently or make sexual overtures, not only to his spouse, but sometimes to inappropriate people such as strangers or other family members. It is thought that some of this behavior may be a desire on the patient's part for reassurance and comfort.

At the end, the victim cannot attend to the simplest details of daily life and may not be able to recognize his spouse or even himself in the mirror!

Another typical case history is that of Arthur, a professor at a well-known university. He was renowned for his fine lectures and many published works. Around the age of sixty he started forgetting the names of his colleagues and students. Initially, this was mildly amusing to the students and moderately confusing to his colleagues. Then he would forget to turn up for lectures, or if he did, he would lose his train of thought and repeat himself. His behavior was no longer amusing or simply confusing to either his students or colleagues. Finally, he had to retire. He tried to write articles at home, but soon, this proved too much for him. Writing became very laborious as he would forget what it was he wanted to say or which words to use.

His wife tried to keep up their normal routine of frequent outings to the theater, concerts, and restaurants, times that had brought them joy all their life. But it was embarrassing when Arthur would forget where he was and jump up to leave in the middle of a performance, or when he went to the men's room and forgot the way back to his seat.

Gradually, Arthur could not be permitted to go anywhere on his own. He also lost the ability to dress properly, putting on his pajamas to go out, or a shirt and tie to sleep in. A few minutes after eating he would forget that he had had his meal and demand to know when it would be served. He had difficulty in using cutlery, making it necessary for his wife to spoon-feed him. Mealtimes became a nightmare as Arthur would wander away from the dining table before he had finished. At night he was restless, unable to sleep, and he had to be watched in case he wandered outside and got lost. Personal hygiene became a task beyond his capabilities, but he violently disliked being bathed, groomed, and taken to the bathroom by others, even his wife.

Looking after Arthur was more than a full-time job and, despite professional assistance, his wife finally made the painful decision to put Arthur in a nursing home where she thought he would be better cared for and safe.

The progression of the disease is continuous but some patients may deteriorate more rapidly than others. In some, the disease can be full-blown within a year, while in others it may take several decades to reach the same stage. The average duration of the illness is around ten to twelve years.

## Is All Senility Caused by Alzheimer's Disease?

It is estimated that Alzheimer's is responsible for one-half of all the dementias that develop in later life. But it is definitely not just a natural part of aging; it is an *abnormal* pathological process.

The other 50 percent of cases of dementia is due to various causes. One major cause is damage to the brain tissue; it is referred to as "multi-infarct dementia" (MID). MID is the result of blockages of the cerebral blood vessels caused by multiple small strokes, resulting in a reduction in the volume of active brain tissue.

MID is different from Alzheimer's disease in that its onset is much more abrupt, and it may be characterized by periods of remission and sudden worsening—in contrast to the steady progression of Alzheimer's.

The symptoms of MID are also more variable, depending on which part of the brain is affected. Heart disease, angina, atherosclerosis, high blood pressure, diabetes mellitus, obesity, and cigarette smoking are all risk factors in the development of MID.

About fifteen percent of the dementias in later life are multi-infarct dementias. Another 25 percent are due to a combination of the above and Alzheimer's disease. The remaining 10 percent are due to such causes as:

1. Psychiatric depression. Depression occurs commonly in the elderly due to changing social, economic, and emotional circumstances. Although not a true dementia, it may result in eating and sleeping disturbances, anxiety, social withdrawal, memory loss, and intellectual impairment.
2. Some types of Parkinson's disease. These may result in marked mental deterioration.
3. Normal pressure hydrocephalus (NPH). Various conditions such as tumors, hemorrhages, and injury can block the drainage of the fluid in the brain into the general circulation and cause NPH, resulting in a gradual dementia and other neurological signs.
4. Infectious, traumatic, nutritional, chemical, metabolic, and hereditary causes.

And, of course, the causes of some dementias are still unknown.

Alzheimer's disease cannot be definitely diagnosed except after death upon examination of the brain of its victim, but a diagnosis of the illness can be made based on *excluding* other known causes and symptoms of dementia, such as those listed above. Often the diagnosis of a patient will involve a number of consultations with several different physicians. A study at the University of Michigan found that most families began recognizing adverse changes in their affected relative about four years prior to a diagnosis of Alzheimer's disease being made. Most of these changes involved memory loss, confusion, disorientation, and personality problems. In the Michigan study, over 60 percent of the cases were originally misdiagnosed two or more times.

(Should the abnormal protein "ALZ-50 antigen," discovered in mid-1986 in the brains of Alzheimer's patients, eventually be detectable in cerebrospinal fluid, it will become a relatively direct procedure to test for the presence of this unique protein and, hence, to diagnose Alzheimer's disease with certainty while the patient is alive.)

## What Are the Physiological Effects of Alzheimer's Disease?

### 1.) In the Deceased

On autopsy, it has been found that there are three major changes within the brains of Alzheimer's suffers—double strands of neurofibrillary tangles, senile plaques, and granulovacular degeneration—which seem to be associated with increased mental impairment.

The neurofibrillary tangles (abnormal fibers within the cell) are found mainly in the cerebral cortex (a thin layer of nerve cell bodies that forms the outermost part of the cerebrum), especially in the area thought to be associated with short-term memory and the emotions. Although the number of tangles increases in all persons with advancing age, sufferers of Alzheimer's disease show a much higher density of these tangles. In addition, the mineral aluminum bound with silicates seems to be specifically concentrated in these tangles, giving the brains of Alzheimer's victims a much higher-than-normal level of aluminum.

Secondly, senile plaques (concentrations of decayed neural material) are also found in increased numbers in Alzheimer's victims. They are usually found in the same areas of the brain as are the tangles.

Thirdly, abnormal changes within the cells are found in greater concentrations in Alzheimer's sufferers, in the same areas within the brain as the other two changes.

Chemical changes have also been found in the brains of Alzheimer's victims. The production of one important neurotransmitter (a chemical necessary for communication between nerves), acetylcholine, has been found to be deficient in those areas where the physical changes noted above have been identified. The result of those physical and chemical changes is that the flow of information within the brain is disjointed and halted.

Studies have also shown that the blood flow to the brain is reduced in persons with Alzheimer's disease, particularly in the same areas where the other changes have taken place. (Later on we will see how a novel treatment, termed "chelation," may improve blood flow and diminish symptoms.)

The brains of Alzheimer's victims also change in shape. The outer layers degenerate, especially in the area of the forehead and inside the temples.

2.) In the Living

Another finding in Alzheimer's sufferers is chromosomal damage and loss of white blood cells, which make up the body's immune system. It has been found that the higher the number of abnormal body cells of these types, the lower the individual's performance on a series of psychological tests of intellectual functioning.

## Who Gets Alzheimer's Disease?

The number of cases of Alzheimer's disease is difficult to quantify because of the problems of misdiagnosis and overlap with other conditions, such as depression and overmedication (two serious problems in the elderly). Very probably, however, the incidence of the condition is underestimated.

An Alzheimer's-type dementia has been known as far back as ancient Greece, but it is impossible to estimate in what numbers, in which groups, or over what areas it has occurred throughout history. But there are patterns to this disease worth considering.

## Is Alzheimer's Disease Hereditary?

Alzheimer's disease appears to run in families. Immediate ("first-order") relatives of a patient with the disease have a great risk of developing the disorder themselves. But the incidence of the disease as it occurs in both identical and fraternal sets of twins, though somewhat elevated, is not convincingly high enough to "prove" a hereditary link. It is thought that the disease may be inherited in some families as an autosomal (any chromosome other than those that determine the sex) dominant gene (that is, the gene located on a non-sex chromosome) and may appear in 50 percent of the offspring.

It has been found in a number of studies that in the families of patients with Alzheimer's disease, there is a slightly increased association with Down's syndrome. This evidence further emphasizes the significance of a possible genetic predisposition in the development of Alzheimer's disease. This predisposition, taken together with an aluminum overload and serious nutritional deficits, may induce the disease process.

It is people with Alzheimer's disease in their immediate relatives for whom this risk-reduction program is especially valuable.

Cases of Alzheimer's disease that occur without a clear family history may represent a separate form of the disease. Compared to age-matched controls, however, patients with non-familial Alzheimer's disease still showed the characteristic and severe neuron damage seen in familial Alzheimer's disease.

The percentage of cases of Alzheimer's disease that can be attributed to the familial form is not clear, but estimates range from 10 percent to 60 percent of all cases. A U.S. Government Information Paper, published in January 1984, suggests that if all four grandparents of an individual live to the age of seventy-five, "the chances are better than 50 percent," that one grandparent would be affected by the disease. They conclude that "almost all of us will have an affected relative or close family friend."

Alzheimer's disease is thought to be responsible for half of all the dementias that occur in later life. It is also responsible for half of all admissions to nursing homes and long-term care mental hospitals.

To reduce symptoms in only 20 percent of patients, those for whom this risk-reduction program may prove effective, would return the gift of productive, even enjoyable, life to nearly five hundred thousand people.

For those of us in our forties and fifties who want to reduce the risk of this disease, *reducing* aluminum and *adding* chelating nutrients and other nutrients that permit choline to activate nerve transmission efficiently may be the single most important dietary change we ever make. We will discuss this in more detail in chapters six and seven.

# 3

# WHAT CAUSES ALZHEIMER'S DISEASE?

Theories abound regarding the "cause" of Alzheimer's disease.[1] Some say that it is caused by a "slow" virus (so called because the symptoms appear only after a prolonged incubation period of about eighteen months), by bacteria, by toxic metals (aluminum and lead), that it is genetically inherited, or that it is due to immune system malfunction.

None of these theories has been proven, and no one of them alone can explain the full clinical picture, including the anatomical and biological changes seen in the disease.

Out of the confusion and despair, some very encouraging leads to the cause of Alzheimer's disease have been uncovered. On autopsy, a specific region of the brains of Alzheimer's victims has been found to contain a much higher-than-normal level of aluminum. Aluminum appears to be specifically con-

1 This discussion is based, in part, on the excellent review article by Richard J. Wurtman that appeared in Scientific American (January 1985). References cited in this chapter may be found in Dr. Wurtman's professional publication listed in my bibliography.

centrated in the tangled double strands of nerve fibers—the neurofibrillary tangles—that are markers of the disease and are prominently found in the cerebral cortex.

The cause(s) of such specific nerve cell degeneration is not yet precisely known. But, in a genetically predisposed person, any number of factors might cause such brain damage. As we have seen, this defect seems to run in families, with genes and environmental factors playing their roles. But additional events must occur to trigger "disease."

Possible events include viral or bacterial infection; endocrine system failure; a defect in metabolism; or cardiovascular problems. Injury, low brain oxygen, and toxins, including metals such as aluminum, are also suspected.

While the evidence is strong that aluminum is a key culprit for many people who are particularly sensitive to this ubiquitous metal, owing to a long-standing mineral imbalance, it is necessary and important that we also look at *all* of the above possible links to this frightful disease.

## Viral Infection

There is a possibility that viral agents may be involved in the development of Alzheimer's disease. Evidence from other uncommon dementias in man and animals that are transmissible by virus supports this premise.

The following four illnesses exhibiting dementia have been found to be caused by infectious viral agents, called "slow viruses" because the diseases have a long incubation period before the overt appearance of symptoms.

*Kuru.* This illness is found among certain New Guinea tribes. Victims develop disturbances in walking, speech, and other movements, and intellectual function diminishes. Death, usually due to secondary infections, occurs within four months to two years after the onset of the disease. Strangely, about eighty percent of the adults who contract the disease are women—and children are also affected. It has been found that in the particular tribes that are affected, cannibalism is practiced.

The women and children eat the brains of the cannibalized victims while the men in the tribe eat the other parts of the body. So the illness appears to be induced by a virus carried in diseased brains. In confirmation of this theory, scientists have been able to develop the disease in chimpanzees by inoculating them with infected brain tissue.

*Scrapie*. This is a disease causing neurological disorders and death in sheep and goats. It has been transferred by inoculation into mice, who develop a similar disease.

*Mink encephalopathy*. This is a neurological illness that occurs in minks, but it is thought that the minks contract the disease by eating the carcasses of scrapie-infected sheep.

*Creutzfeldt-Jakob disease* (*CJD*). This is a dementia found in man, which, like kuru, can be produced in chimpanzees by inoculation with infected human brain tissue.

The above conditions progress slowly but steadily, as does Alzheimer's disease. The structures and twisted filaments found in the brains of animals and people with these diseases are *not* present in Alzheimer's disease. But, according to Dr. Wurtman, "They do share some immunological properties with the amyloid fibrils of neurofibrillary tangles."

To see whether similar factors operate in Alzheimer's disease, scientists have tried to inject different animals with brain tissue removed from Alzheimer's patients after death.

These patients had a strong family history of dementia and developed the disease early, in their forties and fifties. Several species of monkeys have been found to develop neurological disorders (but *not* Alzheimer's disease), two to four years after inoculation.

## Inadequate Oxygenation of the Brain

It has been hypothesized that an inadequate flow of blood to the brain due to a vascular problem (commonly referred to as poor circulation and hardening of the arteries), can, over a period of time, impair mental function and may be involved in the etiology of Alzheimer's disease. As mentioned in chapter two, atherosclerosis and other conditions that affect blood supply are risk factors in the development of multi-infarct dementia, another cause of senility. However, treatment of Alzheimer's patients in hyper-baric oxygen chambers, or with drugs to increase tissue oxygenation, has not improved intellectual performance. This is because other factors are involved with Alzheimer's disease.

Richard S. J. Frackowiak and J. M. Gibbs of the National Hospital for Nervous Diseases in London have reported some interesting findings (*Scientific American*, January 1985). Between the ages of thirty-three and sixty-one, most people have a decrease of blood flow to the brain. In an effort to make up for this deficit, the brain utilizes a larger amount of oxygen from the blood.

Patients with senility (not of the Alzheimer's variety) have been found to have a reduced cerebral blood flow and cerebral metabolic rate of oxygen and glucose. Other findings also indicate abnormal protein metabolism and reduced levels of protein synthesis in the brains of persons with dementia.

In addition, patients with non-Alzheimer's type of senility have been found to have a reduced tolerance to glucose, when compared with nondiabetic controls and persons with cerebrovascular disease, indicating that the disease may not be confined solely to the brain but may be more widespread.

Alzheimer's patients, by comparison, suffer an even *greater* decrease of blood flow to the brain, but the brain does not compensate by taking more oxygen from the blood. Instead, the blood flow and oxygen consumption of Alzheimer's patients declines to approximately 30 percent below that of other aged people not suffering from dementia.

Other studies show a similar decline in the rate at which the brain consumes glucose, the brain's major source of energy.

Dr. Frank Benson, of the University of California at Los Angeles School of Medicine, reported (*Scientific American*, January 1985) findings that support those of the physicians from London. He reported that it was found in Alzheimer's patients that the brain consumed from 30 percent to 50 percent less glucose in each of the four cortical regions of the brain, and in one subcortical region, in patients whose dementia had resulted from several small strokes. He further stated that the glucose deficit seemed to be confined to the regions of the brain affected by the strokes suffered.

Further support of this evidence was reported by John P. Blass, of the Cornell University Medical College (*Scientific American*, January 1985). Upon examination, brain and skin cell samples of Alzheimer's patients showed a deficiency in the enzyme phosphofructokinase, an enzyme necessary for converting glucose to high-energy compounds. With the damage to the brain cells of Alzheimer's victims, a decrease in the number of cells consuming oxygen would be expected to lower the brain's demand for blood. Yet, from the observation of scientists, the reduced blood flow is much lower than could be accounted for by the loss of such brain cells.

Arnold B. Scheinbel, of the UCLA School of Medicine, has noted (*Scientific American*, January 1985) that the dilation and contraction of arterioles is particularly lessened in the brains of patients suffering from dementia. These actions are controlled by small neurons and, when diminished, suggest diminished nerve function.

It is hypothesized that the loss of nerves (such as the damage seen in the neurofibrillary tangles of Alzheimer's victims' brains) controlling the blood flow lessens the flow of oxygen-rich blood to brain cells.

## Metabolic Factors

Normally, the level of cortisonelike compounds increases with age, but even *higher* levels have been found in the blood of patients with degenerative senility, including Alzheimer's, and may play a role in its pathology. These compounds have been found to influence enzymes in a critical brain system, but the exact consequences of this effect are still largely speculative.

## Abnormal Regulation of Calcium Within the Nerve Cell

Because calcium is essential for the release of neurotransmitters and for the utilization of glucose by nerve cells, it has been hypothesized that a defect in calcium uptake, as seen in patients with Alzheimer's disease, is due to a problem in the regulation of calcium within the nerve cell. Such a defect in calcium regulation also develops in heart cells with age.

## Autoimmunity

It is known that a toxin (such as aluminum) or a virus might cause autoimmune reactions to occur. Changes produced in brain cells may cause the body's immune system to think that foreign cells are present and marshal a "self-against-self" reaction against the damaged nerve fibers, similar to what happens in an allergic reaction elsewhere in the body.

Brain autoantibodies have been found circulating in old (but not young) animals and may represent a breakdown in the membrane that normally separates the blood and brain. This membrane normally keeps the antibodies separate from the brain antigens.

The level of brain antibodies in the blood of patients with dementia is significantly higher than in age-matched controls without dementia. It may be that aluminum increases the permeability of the membrane separating blood and brain.

## Malnutrition

It has been suggested that an inadequate intake over years of various nutrients essential to health can predispose the body to the development of Alzheimer's disease. This subject is of great importance and will be explored in more detail in the last chapter.

## Genetic Factors

As mentioned earlier, there is an increased risk of Alzheimer's disease in close relatives of a patient with the disease. However, other events may be needed to "trigger" the disease.

A study by Leonard L. Heston, of the University of Minnesota Medical School, following his observation of the parents, siblings, and second-degree relatives of 125 deceased patients of confirmed Alzheimer's disease, reported that 87 of the relatives developed a dementing illness. Of the 87 relatives, in all autopsied cases the dementia was diagnosed as Alzheimer's disease.

Down's syndrome patients who survive past the age of forty have an unusually high incidence of an Alzheimer's-like disease. An autopsy *on* these patients showed neurofibrillary tangles and senile plaques, identical to those seen in Alzheimer's disease.

If genetics is a factor in Alzheimer's disease, how does a genetic error (the term "genetic" implies "from the moment of conception") remain hidden for so many years? This is not an unknown phenomenon. Certain other diseases, such as Huntington's disease, are known to remain dormant through the first few decades of life, not striking the victims until they are in their prime of life.

Doubt is thrown on the genetic factor *alone* being a cause for Alzheimer's disease because of the variations of the age of onset in identical twins. First symptoms of dementia in one set of identical twins were thirteen years apart. As twins are known to have identical genes, this suggests that environmental or metabolic factors must play a part in determining the onset of Alzheimer's disease.

The recent discovery of the gene for amyloid by a scientist at the National Institutes of Health does little to confirm the genetic basis of Alzheimer's disease. All this discovery confirms is that the genetic *potential* for developing this abnormal protein exists in each of us. Environmental factors obviously must operate for this disease process to occur. These factors include a lifetime deficiency of calcium and magnesium, other nutritional defects, and an excessive intake of aluminum and other toxic metals.

## What About Aluminum?

One composite theory that could possibly explain each of the above theories is that the onset of Alzheimer's disease is due to a complex nutritional imbalance and that in a large number of sensitive individuals the intake of aluminum from external sources is further *implicated.* Since aluminum will normally be excreted by healthy people who have adequate intakes of calcium and magnesium, this toxic metal hypothesis also lends itself to an overall nutritional hypothesis.

Alzheimer's disease has not been around forever. Nor have aluminum cans, foil, or aluminum-saturated drugs, foods, or drinks. Unlike some bizarre notions of health and disease, the connection between this disease and aluminum and other nutritional factors is overwhelmingly strong. Not yet proof positive, but strong enough to warrant our concern; strong enough that scientific papers continue to appear reaffirming this connection (see the bibliography at the back of this book). In short, the "Aluminum Connection" is strong enough that you cannot afford the risk of ignoring it and of not making those few changes that may save you from a second half of your life as a mental vegetable.

Remember this, even if you read what follows and remain skeptical: you will not be able to find many biomedical researchers who will argue that aluminum is good for you! It is neurotoxic, damaging to the nervous system, even in minute quantities. You simply do not want it in your body and in your brain.

What is the evidence?

## Aluminum Toxicity in the Brain

There is considerable evidence, in both experimental animals and man, implicating a disorder of aluminum metabolism in Alzheimer's disease.

Daniel Perl at the University of Vermont College of Medicine, and D. R. Crapper McLachlan at the University of Toronto have both reported higher concentrations of aluminum in the brains of Alzheimer's victims after death, particularly concentrated in one of the pathological areas of the disease, the neurofibrillary tangle. In experimental aluminum encephalopathy in cats and rabbits, toxic concentrations of aluminum were found in the brain tissue in formations resembling the neurofibrillary tangles of Alzheimer's disease. Although the aluminum was concentrated in several different areas in the animals' brains, in both man and the animals the aluminum was found in the same part of the cell: that is, within the nucleus in association with the DNA-containing structures.

As mentioned in chapter two, Alzheimer's is a progressive disease causing loss of mental functions over a number of years. It starts with memory loss, but slowly all other aspects of intellectual function deteriorate, leading ultimately to a state of "vegetation." Motor disorders, including spasms and jerks, and seizures also develop.

In cats and rabbits a toxic dose of aluminum injected into the brain causes a progressive encephalopathy, with death resulting from seizures similar to Alzheimer's disease. Although the time span of the experimental disease in the animals is very short (between fourteen to twenty-eight days), the course the disease follows is the same as in Alzheimer's disease.

From these experiments we can conclude that the manifestation of aluminum toxicity does not necessarily depend on an aged or deteriorating nervous system. Other species of animals, such as rats, mice, and certain monkeys are resistant to aluminum toxicity, and it is thought that susceptibility to the metal may be influenced by genetic factors.

Further evidence as to the involvement of aluminum toxicity in a brain disorder related to Alzheimer's disease comes from Guam, the Kii Peninsula of Japan, and Western New Guinea, where there is an unusually high incidence of amyotrophic lateral sclerosis (ALS) and parkinsonism associated with severe dementia (PD).

In these conditions, neurofibrillary degeneration with increased aluminum concentrations, as found in Alzheimer's disease, occurs, although the aluminum is found in both the cytoplasm and nucleus of the neurons. Senile plaques do not develop. Higher concentrations of aluminum are seen in all the affected tissue of the victims compared to age-matched controls.

It has been found that in the soil and water of these areas, there are relatively *high levels* of *aluminum* and manganese, and extremely low levels of *calcium* and *magnesium*! Other evidence, from a number of victims in Guam, indicates that they were deprived of adequate amounts of calcium and magnesium in their early years. All this suggests that aluminum may be used as a substitute for calcium by the body, or it may enter the brain via the same transport mechanism as calcium. Of course, in these geographical areas, genetic and other environmental factors may also play a role in the development of aluminum toxicity.

An interpretation of these data by experts is in order. According to F. Yoshimasu, Department of Neuropsychiatry, Wakayama Medical College, Japan, "Recent studies, however, have shown that aluminum is implicated in certain human central nervous system (CNS) diseases including Alzheimer's disease and the dialysis encephalopathy syndrome." (In Chen and Yase, 1984, p. 357.)

Dr. H. N. Wisniewski and coworkers of the New York State Institute of Basic Research in Developmental Disabilities conclude and state, from the above observations, "The tentative conclusion reached from these results is that the pathogenesis of ALS, PD, and premature occurrence of PHF [paired helical filaments], in neurologically normal people in this region, may include environmental factors, especially the high natural abundance of aluminum."

In Alzheimer's disease, while the brain shows elevated levels of aluminum, other body fluids and organs, including blood and cerebral spinal fluid, do not exhibit similarly high levels of the mineral. In fact, in one study, patients with dementia were found to have abnormally low levels of aluminum in the cerebral spinal fluid. In addition, as mentioned above, in Alzheimer's disease, the aluminum is concentrated in the region of the nucleus of the nerve cells.

In contrast, in a type of dementia brought about by kidney dialysis (discussed in chapter four), in which victims were subjected to a chronic overload of aluminum (through medication and the tap water used for dialysis), aluminum was concentrated in the cytoplasm of the cell. But there were no signs of neurologic damage until levels were ten to twenty times greater than normal.

This dialysis dementia manifests itself with speech difficulties, which progress over a period of months, and include tremor, memory loss, and personality changes. In extreme cases, patients who suffer from this syndrome will eventually lose their motor coordination, their speech, and very often will experience seizures, followed by death.

Normally, the brain is protected from toxic substances by the blood-brain barrier, a membrane. However, because excess aluminum is concentrated in brain tissue in Alzheimer's victims, it is hypothesized that in this disease state, there exists a defect in this barrier system, allowing the aluminum to enter brain cells.

Sometimes though, in kidney failure or in cases of stroke or a severe brain concussion, this blood-brain barrier is damaged, and toxic substances in the blood may enter the brain. We see this occurring in patients who rely on high quantities of aluminum-containing antacids. These people have high concentrations of aluminum in their blood. In the event of a physical blow, or if they are undergoing dialysis owing to kidney failure, a toxic reaction due to the aluminum occurs in the brain, producing severe seizures.

Surprisingly, even high concentrations of sugar in our diet may open up the blood-brain barrier! Experimentally this has been demonstrated in animals (*Scientific American,* September 1986). When we take a glucose-tolerance test, we become dizzy after ingesting a large glassful of a glucose solution. This is most likely a result of the sugar crossing the blood-brain barrier. Such an easy pathway into the brain may permit the entry of aluminum and other toxic metals.

It is important to note though, that the aluminum that penetrates the blood-brain barrier does not enter the cytoplasm of cells, but instead, enters the nucleus and gains access to the DNA-containing structures there (that is, the chromosomes or genetic material). Thus, there may be some initial pathogenic event causing damage to the blood-brain barrier or altering the metabolism of aluminum in the brain, permitting this metal to participate in neuronal damage.

Dr. Wisniewski concludes from the above, "All of the evidence points to the requirement of high levels of aluminum in the brain as being necessary for the development of dialysis dementia, even though it may not be the direct cause."

"Although the recent reports from ALS and PD cases in the western Pacific region provide evidence that the role of aluminum in encephalopathy is still an open question, the studies with dialysis dementia and aluminum-treated animals provide strong evidence that high levels of aluminum in the brain are associated with neurological dysfunction, including disturbances in cognitive functions. It is clear that under some circumstances, aluminum is a neurotoxic substance and that we need to know more about its mechanism of action before we can determine with certainty its role in disease, and the conditions in which it may be hazardous." (Wisniewski, 1985).

At the moment, the evidence is not conclusive enough as to whether aluminum is a primary *cause* of Alzheimer's disease or whether its accumulation is a *consequence* of other disease factors. Nevertheless, for the reasons outlined in this chapter and elsewhere in this book, we must be cautious of this metal and avoid ingesting it so far as is possible.

## Abnormal Production of Brain Signal-Transmitting Chemicals

Choline is a vitamin like molecule that is essential to numerous functions in the human body. It is a component of cell membranes and is also a constituent of a type of phospholipid found in high concentrations in the brain. Choline is also a component of acetylcholine, which functions in transmitting nerve impulses. Normally, choline can be synthesized by the body, but sometimes deficiencies arise.

For this nutrient to be made within the body, the amino acid methionine is required. In addition, folic acid and vitamin B-12 are required for its synthesis. A good, mixed diet generally provides enough of the starting materials to permit synthesis of choline. However, people who have lived on severely protein-deficient diets that are overly rich in highly refined foods may often experience a choline deficiency.

It has recently been found that aluminum can inhibit the transportation of choline within brain cells. It also inhibits the action of an enzyme known as choline acetyltransferase (also known as CAT), which is an enzyme that manufactures acetylcholine in brain cells. These findings have led some scientists to believe that aluminum may, in part, contribute to the cholinergic nerve cell deficits observed in Alzheimer's disease.

The most obvious change in the signal-transmitting chemicals found in the brain of patients with Alzheimer's disease is a 40 percent to 90 percent decrease in the quantities of the enzyme CAT. This enzyme is found both in the cerebral cortex and the hippocampus regions of the brain. CAT is severely reduced in Alzheimer's patients, even during the first year the symptoms appear.

It is clinically important to note that objective tests of mental function show a strong negative change as this critical enzyme, CAT, is lost. Further, when healthy young volunteers were subjected to injections of scopalomine, which is a drug that destroys choline activity, temporary confusion and memory loss was observed, resembling the early symptoms of Alzheimer's disease.

This biochemical theory was first clearly put forth in 1976 by two groups of scientists. The leaders were Peter Davies, of The University of Edinburgh, Faculty of Medicine, and David Bowan, of the Institute of Neurology, in London.

These men reported that the level of the enzyme CAT, which helps in the uptake of choline, is often reduced up to 90 percent in Alzheimer's disease patients. More specifically, the enzyme CAT helps speed the synthesis of acetylcholine from its starter compounds, choline and acetyl coenzyme A. As this CAT enzyme is lost, cholinergic- or acetylcholine-releasing nerve terminals are also diminished in two specific regions of the brain.

These findings have been confirmed by other scientists, and their significance was recently summarized by Dr. Richard J. Wurtman, of the Massachusetts Institute of Technology, as follows: "It seems to many of us to be the clue most likely eventually to point to the cause of Alzheimer's disease. It also suggests an explanation for the disease's cardinal symptom, loss of memory. It is therefore plausible to hypothesize that some of the cognitive deficits of Alzheimer's disease are the direct result of a reduction in the acetylcholine mediator transmission of nerve impulses."

This hypothesis of restoring the level of the enzyme CAT or of restoring the activity of choline leads to a belief that a drug, or substance that could restore the level of acetylcholine, might in fact, be effective in treating Alzheimer's disease.

This is based, in part, on the success of treating Parkinson's disease by adding back the neurotransmitter dopamine. This is achieved by use of the drug L-Dopa. While the use of drugs has had mixed results, trials with choline and lecithin, which are the precursors of acetylcholine, have offered very promising results. A carefully constructed, long-term, and well-controlled study of the effect of purified lecithin added to the diets has recently been reported by Drs. Adrienne Little and Raymond Levy, of Kings College Hospital, London. They reported significant and continuing improvement in the behavior of eight out of twenty-four people with Alzheimer's disease. Interestingly, the eight people who responded to this cholinergic therapy were approximately ten years older than those who did not improve.

Perhaps the most significant findings of this study are that lecithin preparations must be highly pure (containing near 90 percent phosphatidylcholine) and that *moderate*, but precise, doses are required for beneficial effects.

This leads some workers in the field to speculate that there are several types of Alzheimer's disease and that people who contract the disease later on in life tend to have a milder form of the illness, where the effects largely occur in neurons involved in choline transport. While we do not know precisely why levels of CAT are reduced in Alzheimer's disease, recent experiments have shown that aluminum can inhibit choline transport when studied in rat brain nerve endings and also when studied in human red blood cells. Our erythrocytes, or red blood cells, possess a choline transport system that has several functional properties similar to those in our nerve cell uptake system. These studies indicate that aluminum can significantly inhibit the transportation of choline.

Later on, when we discuss the nutritional treatment of Alzheimer's, we will see how associated nutrients can help increase the uptake of choline into neurons and also how certain foods that remove aluminum from our brains and other tissues may be of value in preventing and treating this disease.

The above factors are all being explored in an attempt to elucidate the cause and pathology of Alzheimer's disease. While much progress has been made in investigating the chemical and cellular bases of the disease, the exact causes of the degeneration of the brain tissue are not known. It is hoped, however, that by correcting the pathological processes, the disease can be halted or alleviated.

It seems that some combination of processes involving toxic (i.e. aluminum), infectious, genetic, or other factors (perhaps including age-related changes), may impair neuronal function leading to the characteristic damage seen in Alzheimer's disease. By utilizing nutritional and drug therapy we can counteract these processes in some patients, as we will see in chapters six and seven.

# PART II

# Solutions

# 4

# REDUCING ALUMINUM

Now we know what Alzheimer's disease is and that any of us could be a potential victim. We have examined the pathology of the disease and the latest theories being explored. With improper nutrition considered as a potential contributing factor of Alzheimer's disease, and the presence of the higher-than-normal levels of aluminum in the brains of Alzheimer's victims, it seems prudent that a risk-reduction program be outlined.

## Other Diseases Associated with Excess Aluminum

Besides Alzheimer's disease, other human diseases have been associated with higher-than-normal concentrations of aluminum in various bodily tissues. While it is well known that "observable pathology does not necessarily account for a disorder," aluminum is at best, nonessential, at worst, toxic. This is *further* inducement for eliminating the metal from our foods, medicines, and cookware.

1. *PULMONARY DISEASES.* A distinctive type of pulmonary fibrosis with emphysema has been seen in workers exposed to high levels of powdered aluminum metal, as in the manufacture of aluminum abrasives.

2. The inhalation of aluminum dust in other industries has also resulted in the development of lung diseases among the workers, leading in some cases to death. As early as 1962, a case of pulmonary fibrosis was described with accompanying encephalopathy, and it was realized for the first time that aluminum could accumulate in the brain tissues.

3. *BONE DISEASE.* Aluminum has various effects on bone formation and maintenance. A high dietary intake of aluminum (for example, when antacids are used frequently) has been found to increase the excretion of calcium in the urine and increase the excretion of phosphate in the feces (by binding with it in the gut). This often results in bone demineralization and may possibly lead to osteomalacia (a metabolic bone disease resulting from vitamin D deficiency, commonly called "rickets" in children) and osteoporosis (a decrease in bone tissue mass, resulting in crush fractures from minimal or no trauma). Both calcium and phosphate are needed for proper bone formation. Aluminum may also accumulate in bone tissue and inhibit normal calcification there.

4. Many patients with kidney disease who are on hemodialysis (in which an artificial kidney is used

to filter the blood) have been found to develop a type of bone disease called "renal osteodystrophy," which is characterized by bone pain; aching, weak muscles; and fracturing. The bones of these patients have higher concentrations than normal of aluminum. This is attributed to the use of tap water containing aluminum in dialysis and treatment with antacids containing aluminum. This bone disease can develop despite normal levels of calcium and phosphate in the blood of these patients.

5. In conclusion, it appears that chronic exposure to higher-than-normal levels of aluminum is toxic to bone metabolism in everyone, but those with impaired kidney function may be much more sensitive to aluminum toxicity and at greater risk.

6. *DIALYSIS ENCEPHALOPATHY.* Many kidney patients on hemodialysis were also found to develop a type of progressive fatal brain disease (encephalopathy), characterized by impaired speech, dementia, and seizures. Their brains were found to have elevated levels of aluminum, but in most cases, there were no other specific changes as found in Alzheimer's disease. There was also no evidence of a "slow virus" being at work because injection of the diseased brain tissue into monkeys did not produce any symptoms of encephalopathy after three and a half years.

7. *ANEMIA.* Further evidence of the toxicity of high doses of aluminum comes from the development of a certain type of anemia in kidney patients on

hemodialysis. This is a severe anemia and is found in patients with abnormally high levels of the mineral in their blood. Their levels of hemoglobin (the iron-containing pigment in the blood) drop to very low values despite adequate supplements of iron and other nutrients necessary for hemoglobin formation. The anemia has been found to be reversible after the aluminum is removed from the dialysis water. It is speculated that the presence of aluminum in the bone interferes with the synthesis of hemoglobin, which takes place in the bone marrow.

8. *GASTRIC DISORDERS.* It appears that the use of aluminum-containing antacids in normal persons delays the emptying of the stomach into the intestines by decreasing the contractions of the stomach muscles. In addition, such antacids can cause severe constipation by again inhibiting muscle contraction in the intestines. An aluminum overload can also cause flatulence, inflammation, and colitis.

9. Kidney patients on hemodialysis have been found to develop anorexia (loss of appetite), vomiting, and weight loss when subjected to high levels of aluminum.

10. *CARDIOTOXICITY.* An enzyme critical to the proper functioning of the heart has been found to be inhibited by aluminum (perhaps by depleting the heart muscle of magnesium, which activates this enzyme). Since sudden cardiac death has been linked with a shortage of magnesium in the heart,

it is thought that high levels of aluminum may be toxic to the heart. In kidney patients on hemodialysis who have developed encephalopathy, sudden cardiac deaths have also been noted.

11. *LIVER TOXICITY.* Increased levels of aluminum can accumulate in and damage liver cells, thus impairing liver function. An examination after death of a kidney dialysis patient revealed aluminum present in high concentrations in the liver cells.
12. *BLADDER CANCER.* It has been found that workers exposed to aluminum emissions had a higher risk of bladder cancer, especially if they also smoked.

Higher-than-normal intakes of aluminum have also been linked with sclerosis, nephritis, alcohol dementia, and in children, hyperactivity and psychosis.

Clearly, aluminum toxicity can adversely affect many different systems in your body. A reduction in your overall intake of aluminum may be important in decreasing the risk not only of Alzheimer's disease but also of many other serious and potentially life-threatening conditions.

*What about the abnormal protein found in the brains of Alzheimer's patients?* The recent discovery of an abnormal protein, designated ALZ-50 antigen, in the brains of Alzheimer's disease patients by Drs. Wolozin and Davies of the Albert Einstein College of Medicine, may eventually provide further support for the connection between aluminum and this disease. As you may recall, aluminum and other toxic compounds are normally kept out of our brain tissue by the blood-brain barrier. In the elderly, who have sustained a blow to the head, a stroke, or other head injury, this protective barrier may become somewhat permeable, allowing toxic substances to enter the brain. Aluminum may enter the brain in such cases, possibly stimulating the production of this abnormal protein.

As we learned in the previous chapter, Dr. Peter Davies, one of the same scientists who recently discovered this abnormal protein in the brains of Alzheimer's disease patients, previously discovered that the level of the enzyme CAT, which helps in the uptake of choline, is often reduced up to 90 percent in Alzheimer's disease patients.

Based on these two findings, we may soon learn that aluminum is, in part, responsible both for a decrease in brain levels and functions of the enzyme CAT, as well as in the formation of the abnormal protein ALZ-50 antigen.

This idea is strongly supported, in my opinion, by the findings of a leading researcher in the field, Dr. D. R. Crapper McLachlan, of the Department of Physiology and Medicine, University of Toronto, Canada, who "Suggests that the metal (aluminum), is binding to chromatin, and changes its ability in regard to the initiation of protein synthesis. Conceivably, this might result in the processing of a more or less abnormal protein." (From: Katzman and Terry, *The Neurology of Aging*, p. 72, Philadelphia: F. A. Davis Co., 1983.)

Before we proceed, it is necessary that we understand aluminum and its sources.

### How Does Aluminum Get Into Our Bodies?

Aluminum is a mineral present all around us—in the soil, air, and water. Concentrations in the environment tend to be highly variable due to many factors, including pH (the degree of acidity) and the presence of other substances, and these factors affect its availability to living organisms. Acid rain, for example, causes aluminum to leach out of soil at a higher rate, adding more aluminum to plants and animals in our food chain.

Scientists believe that aluminum is not essential for human health and know that normal levels in the body are quite low. The normal total body content of aluminum in humans is around 30mg. In contrast, high levels of aluminum in the body have been found to be toxic and may play a role in a number of disease conditions, discussed earlier in this chapter, in addition to Alzheimer's disease.

It is estimated that Americans consume around 22-36 milligrams per day of aluminum. In normal, healthy individuals it was thought, until recently, that very little of this was absorbed from the gut and retained in the body. New methods now show that, "As much as 25 percent of some aluminum salts may be absorbed from the gastrointestinal tract" (Lione, 1983). It must also be remembered that your total intake will vary greatly depending on the amount of aluminum in the drinking water and the air in your area, as well as on the types of foods and drugs you consume.

Many scientists now believe that chronic overexposure to aluminum from many sources may lead to an accumulation of too much aluminum in the body's tissue and may result in serious health problems. Some groups in the population may also be at higher risk to these elevated concentrations of aluminum—people with kidney disorders, for example.

How can a concerned individual reduce his intake of aluminum to a low level? By trying to cut down or avoid completely many of the concentrated sources of aluminum! The tables that follow list common sources of this toxic metal in our daily lives. Provided by Dr. Armand Lione of The Associated Pharmacologists and Toxicologists, Washington, D.C., they are published for the first time in a popular book. By reading and applying the information wisely, you should be able to eliminate most aluminum from your life, thereby reducing a key factor in Alzheimer's disease.

It is not easy to eliminate aluminum from your system totally. As we mentioned earlier, it is the most common metal found in the earth's surface, occurring very widely in soils and clays. But through diet, we can greatly decrease the quantity of excess aluminum in our bodies.

By choosing the wrong foods and nonprescription drugs, which contain intentionally added aluminum salts, you can easily increase the daily dietary intake of aluminum ten to one hundred times. People who take large amounts of antacids can sometimes consume as much as five thousand milligrams of added aluminum per day if the antacid is taken as directed! People with rheumatoid arthritis who use aluminum-buffered aspirin as part of their regular drug therapy, may take in as much as seven hundred milligrams of extra aluminum per day.

The first area we want to look at are aluminum-containing *foods and food additives*. While the intake of aluminum from foods may, in some cases, be greater than from drinking water or even antacid tablets, the fiber found in foods slows the rate of absorption of aluminum into the bloodstream. There may not be a great deal of aluminum in most municipal drinking water but what is present is absorbed rapidly, especially on an empty stomach. So, while aluminum in foods may represent a problem, it is not so great a concern as the aluminum found in drinking water and antacids.

## Food and Food Additives

Looking at table 1,[2] you will see that sodium aluminum phosphate is the form of aluminum most frequently used in the United States. In 1970, eighteen million kilograms of sodium aluminum phosphate was used in the American food supply. Some form of this aluminum-containing additive is used to release carbon dioxide gas from baking soda. It is also used to raise self-rising flours, pancake batters, frozen doughs, and cake mixes. When foods prepared from the products that contain sodium aluminum phosphate enter your system, each serving may contain between five and fifteen milligrams of aluminum.

The alkaline aluminum phosphates are used primarily in processed American cheeses. These function as emulsifying agents to produce a cheese that melts easily and has a soft texture. The use of this type of aluminum-containing food additive is most common in the single, individually wrapped, sliced processed cheeses. If alkaline aluminum phosphate is used only at the 3 percent level, one slice of such processed cheese may contain up to 50 milligrams of aluminum!

Another form of this type of food additive is in the sulfate salt form. Here they appear on the product label as "alums." These types of aluminum salts are used as "firming agents" in pickled vegetables and may appear in pickled fruits (such as maraschino cherries). A dill pickle of medium size that has been soaked in a 0.1 percent alum solution may contain between 5 to 10 milligrams of aluminum. This may explain,

2 Tables 1 through 7 are borrowed, with permission, from Dr. Armand Lione's landmark paper, cited in the bibliography as "1985A" and "1985B."

in part, why some of the commercially prepared pickles have a metallic taste.

Sodium aluminum sulfate is typically used in the home as household baking powder. These types of salts were introduced in the United States in baking powders during the 1920s as a replacement for more expensive agents, such as tartaric acid. Such baking powders may contain between 21 percent and 26 percent of their total weight as alum. Therefore, a teaspoon of such a baking powder may contain about 70 milligrams of aluminum. A cake prepared with one to three teaspoons of this baking powder may contain approximately 5 to 15 milligrams of aluminum in each slice.

**Table 1:** Aluminum-Containing Food Additives in the U.S.[3] and Canada[4]

| **Compound** | **% A1** | **total used[5] (kgs)** | **common uses (max. conc.)** | **Al content** |
|---|---|---|---|---|
| Sodium aluminum phosphate | 6.5 (avg) | 18,000,000 | cake mixes, frozen dough, self-rising flour, processed cheese (3–3.5%) | 5–15 mg/serving ~50 mg/slice[6] |
| Sodium aluminum sulfate | 5.9 | 3,600,000 | household baking powders (21–26%) | ~70 mg/tsp ~5 mg/ serving/tsp |
| Aluminum sulfate | 1.3 | 510,000 | food starch modifier | — |

3 U.S. Code of Federal Regulations 21, 182.1125-31, 182.1781, 133.173 ) (1), 182.2727.
4 Canadian Food and Drug Regulations, Division 16, 1981.
5 ~ means "about."
6 ~ means "about."

| | | | | |
|---|---|---|---|---|
| Aluminum ammonium sulfate | 6.0 | 230,000 | pickling salts (0.1%) | — |
| Aluminum potassium sulfate | 5.7 | 3,800 | pickling salts (0.1%) | — |
| Sodium aluminum silicate | 16.0 | n.a. | anticaking agent (2%) | — |

The last category of aluminum-containing food additives is the aluminum silicates. These are used as anticaking agents in nondairy creamers, salt, and other dry, powdered foods and food additives. They may represent up to 2 percent of the final mixture, but since this salt is used in such small amounts in these products, they contribute an insignificant amount of aluminum to your daily intake. (See table 1.)

## Nonprescription Drugs

The next category that we should look at in trying to reduce our overall aluminum intake is the *nonprescription drugs*. The two chief classes of such aluminum-containing drugs are the antacids and the internal analgesics, such as buffered aspirins.

Picking up a bottle of the aluminum-containing antacids, you will see a caution that quotes, "Do not take more than 24 tablets or teaspoonfuls, in a twenty-four-hour period, or use the maximum dosage of this product for more than two weeks." A leading worker in this field of research, Armand Lione, Ph.D., has estimated that such a dosage schedule can deliver between 1,000 and 7,000 milligrams of aluminum per day, should a person take the maximum number of tablets recommended on the product label.

As mentioned previously, the chronic ingestion of aluminum hydroxide and other aluminum salts may greatly increase our overall body load of dietary aluminum. As we have seen, this systemic aluminum is deposited in bone, the parathyroid glands, and the brain. It is unbelievable that millions of women are now being advised to consume antacids as a source of calcium! It is recommended that these products be eliminated, in so far as is possible, from your daily diet.

If women insist on taking calcium supplements, (though skim milk is a far more balanced food source), antacids are *not* the supplement of choice. A tablet combining calcium *with* magnesium is preferred, both because it is free of aluminum and because it contains magnesium, which aids in absorbing calcium.

Table 2, which lists "Aluminum-containing nonprescription drugs" is broken into five categories. The first is antacids, delivering a possible daily dose of 840 to 5,000 milligrams of aluminum. Second are the buffered aspirins, delivering 126 to 728 milligrams of aluminum to systems. Categories three and four are preparations delivering unknown dosages of aluminum to our systems, while category five, "Anti-ulcerative" drugs, may deliver up to 828 milligrams of aluminum each day.

## **Table 2:** Aluminum-Containing Nonprescription Drugs and Sucralfate[7]

| **Drug class** | **Aluminum salts used** | **Aluminum content/ dose† (mg)** | **Possible daily dose Al (mg)** |
|---|---|---|---|
| 1. Antacids | a. aluminum hydroxide | 35–208 | 840–5000 |
| | b. dihydroxyaluminum acetate | 45–72 | |
| | c. aluminum carbonate | n.a. | |
| | d. aluminum oxide | 41 | |
| | e. bismuth aluminate | 55 | |
| | f. magaldrate | 51–61 | |
| | g. dihydroxyaluminum aminoacetate | 100 | |
| | h. dihydroxyaluminum sodium carbonate | 63 | |
| 2. Internal analgesics (buffered aspirins) | aluminum hydroxide<br>b. aluminum glycinate | 9–52<br>10–15 | 126–728 |
| 3. Antidiarrheals | a. kaolin | 120–1450 | |
| | b. aluminum magnesium silicate | 36 | |
| | c. attapulgite | 500–600 | |
| 4. Douches | a. ammonium aluminum sulfate (5–16%) | n.a. | |
| | b. potassium aluminum sulfate | n.a. | |
| | c. "alum" (12%) | n.a. | |
| 5. Anti-ulcerative | a. aluminum sucrose sulfate | 207 | 828 |
| †Single tablet or 5 ml liquid. | | | |

7 Data modified and updated from Penna (1982).

Brand name (manufacturer) for the aluminum salts used in each drug class:

1. Antacids
    a. Albicon (Pfeiffer), AlternaGel (Stuart), Aludrox (Wyeth), Aluminum Hydroxide Gel (Philips Roxane), Alurex (Rexall), Amphojel (Wyeth), A.M.T. (Wyeth), Antacid Powder (DeWitt), Banacid (Buffington), Basaljel Extra Strength (Wyeth), Camalox (Rorer), Creamalin (Winthrop), Delcid (Merrell-Dow), Dialume (Armour), Di-Gel (Plough), Estomul-M (Riker), Flacid (Amfre-Grant), Gaviscon (Marion), Gaviscon-2 (Marion), Gelumina (Amer. Pharm.), Gelusil (Warner-Chilcott), Gelusil II (Warner-Chilcott), Gelusil M (Warner-Chilcott), Glycogel (Central Pharm.), Kessadrox (McKesson), Kolantyl (Merrill-Dow), Kudrox (Kremers-Urban), Liquid Antacid (McKesson), Maalox (Rorer), Maalox No. I (Rorer), Maalox No. 2 (Rorer), Maalox Plus (Rorer), Maalox TC (Rorer), Magna Gel (No. American), Magnatril (Lannett), Mylanta (Stuart), Mylanta II (Stuart), Nephrox (Fleming), Noralac (No. American), Nutrajel (Cenci) Silain-Gel (Robins), Simeco (Wyeth), Syntrogel (Reed & Carnrick), Tempo (Richardson-Vicks), Tralmag (O'Neal, Jones & Feldman), Trimagel (Columbia Medical), Trisogel (Lilly), WinGel (Winthrop).
    b. Aluscop (O'Neal).
    c. Baseljel (Wyeth).
    d. Magnesia and Alumina Oral Suspension (Philips Roxane), Nutramag (Cenci).
    e. Noralac (No. American).
    f. Riopan (Ayerst), Riopan Plus (Ayerst).

   g. Robalate (Robins), Tralmag (O'Neal, Jones & Feldman).
   h. Rolaids (Warner-Lambert).

2. Internal analgesics
   a. Arthritis Pain Formula (Whitehall), Ascriptin (Rorer), Ascriptin A/D (Rorer), B-A (O'Neal, Jones & Feldman), Cama (Dorsey), Cope (Glenbrook), Pabrin (Dorsey), Vanquish Caplet (Glenbrook).
   b. Arthritis Strength Bufferin (Bristol-Myers), Bufferin (Bristol-Myers).

3. Antidiarrheals
   a. Amogel (No. American), Bislad (Central), Diabismul (O'Neal, Jones & Feldman), Dia-eze (Central), Donnagel-PG (Robins), Donnagel (Robins), Kaodene Non-Narcotic (Pfeiffer), Kaodene with Paregoric (Pfeiffer), Kaolin Pectin Suspension (Philips Roxane), Kaopectate (Upjohn), Kaopectate Concentrate (Upjohn), Parepectolin (Rorer), Pargel (Parke-Davis), Pektamalt (Warren-Teed).
   b. Pabisol with Paregoric (Rexall).
   c. Quintese (Lilly), Rheaban (Pfizer).

4. Douches
   a. Massengil Douche Powder (Beecham Products), PMC Douche Powder and Disposable Douche (Thomas & Thompson).
   b. BoCarAl (Beecham Products).
   c. V. A. (Norcliff-Thayer).

5. Anti-ulcerative
   a. Carafate (Marion Labs.).

n.a.—not available.

There are many other drugs available over the counter (called OTC preparations) that contain aluminum. These include clays such as kaolin, which are used for treating diarrhea. These aluminum compounds remain within the gut, absorb moisture and alter the consistency of the stool. Precise absorption of this aluminum has not yet been determined, but these preparations should be used with some caution since we know that aluminum is, in fact, absorbed from the gut in some individuals.

Vaginal douches are another area of concern. Several of these, in fact most that are commercially prepared, do contain aluminum salts (table 3). Some of these compounds are soluble, and possibly absorbed, when applied. To what extent these products are absorbed from the vagina must be determined before their safety can be assured with any certainty.

**Table 3:** Aluminum-Containing Douches[8]

| Brand name (manufacturer) | aluminum salt | concentration |
|---|---|---|
| BoCarAl (Calgon) | potassium aluminum sulfate | n.s. |
| Massengil Douche Powder (Beecham Products) | ammonium aluminum sulfate | n.s. |
| PMC Douche Powder (Thomas & Thompson) | ammonium aluminum sulfate | 16% |
| V.A. (Norcliff-Thayer) | alum | n.s. |
| Summer's Eve (Personal Labs) | potassium aluminum sulfate | n.s. |

n.s.—not specified

Table 4 lists nonprescription *antacids* that contain aluminum, giving their brand name, type of aluminum salt, the concentration of the salt in the tablet, and the approximate

8 Penna (1979)

aluminum content of each particular tablet or teaspoonful, in milligrams. This table should be of particular interest to those who consume antacids on a regular basis. Aluminum intoxication has been shown in some elderly patients who take maintenance doses of such antacids.

As stated earlier and throughout this book, chronic consumption of aluminum-containing antacids and other aluminum-containing nonprescription drugs, may be responsible, in part, for the accumulation of aluminum in the brain cells of Alzheimer's disease patients.

For those who wish to discontinue the ingestion of such antacids, it should be pointed out that there are now more than twenty antacid compounds available that do *not* contain aluminum. These can be found by reading the label of the myriad bottles of antacids in your pharmacy. Those with aluminum must state so under the "ingredients" list.

**Table 4:** Nonprescription Antacids that Contain Aluminum[9]

| | **Brand Name** (manufacturer) | **Aluminum salt** (Concentration) | **Aluminum content/** tablet or tsp. (mg.) |
|---|---|---|---|
| 1. | Albicon (Pfeiffer) | aluminum hydroxide | |
| | tablet | 150 mg | 44 |
| | suspension | 60 mg/ml | 87 |
| 2. | AlternaGel (Stuart) | aluminum hydroxide | |
| | | 120 mg/ml | 174 |
| 3. | Aludrox (Wyeth) | aluminum hydroxide | |
| | tablet | 233 mg | 68 |
| | suspension | 61 mg/ml | 88 |

9 Penna, R.P.: Handbook of Non-prescription Drugs. American Pharmaceutical Assoc., Washington, D.C. 6th ed. 1979. 488 p.

| | | | |
|---|---|---|---|
| 4. | Aluminum Hydroxide Gel | aluminum hydroxide | |
| | (Philips Roxane) | 70 mg/ml | 100 |
| 5. | Alurex (Rexall) | aluminum hydroxide | — |
| | tablet | n.s. | — |
| | suspension | n.s. | — |
| 6. | Aluscop (O'Neal) | dihydroxyaluminum | |
| | capsule | 325 mg | 72 |
| | suspension | 40 mg/ml | 45 |
| 7. | Amphojel (Wyeth) | aluminum hydroxide | |
| | tablet | 300 or 600 mg | 87 or 174 |
| | suspension | 64 mg/ml | 90 |
| 8. | A.M.T. (Wyeth) | aluminum hydroxide | |
| | tablet | 164 mg | 48 |
| | suspension | 61 mg/ml | 88 |
| 9. | Antacid Powder (DeWitt) | aluminum hydroxide | |
| | | 15% | — |
| 10. | Banacid (Buffington) | aluminum hydroxide n.s. | — |
| 11. | Basaljel (Wyeth) | aluminum carbonate n.s. | |
| 12. | Basaljel (Wyeth) | aluminum hydroxide | |
| | Extra Strength | 200 mg/ml | 58 |
| 13. | Camalox (Rorer) | aluminum hydroxide | |
| | tablet | 225 mg | 65 |
| | suspension | 45 mg/ml | 65 |
| 14. | Creamalin (Winthrop) | aluminum hydroxide | |
| | tablet | 248 mg | 72 |
| 15. | Delcid (Merrell-National) | aluminum hydroxide | |
| | suspension | 120 mg | 174 |

| | | |
|---|---|---|
| 16. Dialume (Armour) | aluminum hydroxide | |
| tablet | 500 mg | 145 |
| 17. Di-Gel (Plough) | aluminum hydroxide | |
| tablet | 282 mg | 82 |
| liquid | 56 mg/ml | 82 |
| 18. Estomul-M(Riker) | aluminum hydroxide | |
| tablet | 500 mg | 145 |
| liquid | 184 mg/ml | 265 |
| 19. Flacid (Amfre-Grant) | aluminum hydroxide | |
| tablet | n.s. | — |
| 20. Gelumina (Amer. Pharm.) | aluminum hydroxide | |
| tablet | 250 mg | 72 |
| 21. Gelusil (Warner-Chilcott) | aluminum hydroxide | |
| tablet | 200 mg | 58 |
| suspension | 40 mg/ml | 58 |
| 22. Gelusil II (Warner-Chilcott) | aluminum hydroxide | |
| tablet | 400 mg | 116 |
| suspension | 80 mg/ml | 116 |
| 23. Gelusil M (Warner-Chilcott) | aluminum hydroxide | |
| tablet | 300 mg | 87 |
| suspension | 60 mg/ml | 87 |
| 24. Glycogel (Central Pharm.) | aluminum hydroxide | |
| tablet | 175 mg | 51 |
| 25. Kessadrox (McKesson) | aluminum hydroxide | |
| suspension | 67 mg/ml | 97 |

| | | | |
|---|---|---|---|
| 26. | Kolantyl (Merrell-National) | aluminum hydroxide | |
| | gel | 10 mg/ml | 14 |
| | tablet | 300 mg | 87 |
| | wafer | 180 mg | 52 |
| 27. | Krem (Mallinckrodt) | aluminum hydroxide | |
| | tablet | n.s. | — |
| 28. | Kudrox (Kremers-Urban) | aluminum hydroxide | |
| | tablet | 400 mg | 116 |
| | suspension | 113 mg/ml | 164 |
| 29. | Liquid Antacid (McKesson) | aluminum hydroxide | |
| | suspension | 67 mg/ml | 97 |
| 30. | Maalox (Rorer) | aluminum hydroxide | |
| | #1 tablet | n.s. | — |
| | #2 tablet | n.s. | — |
| | suspension | n.s. | — |
| 31. | Maalox Plus (Rorer) | aluminum hydroxide | |
| | tablet | 200 mg | 58 |
| | suspension | 45 mg/ml | 65 |
| 32. | Magna Gel (No. American) | aluminum hydroxide | |
| | gel | n.s. | — |
| 33. | Magnatril (Lannett) | aluminum hydroxide | |
| | tablet | 260 mg | 75 |
| | suspension | 52 mg/ml | 75 |
| 34. | Maxamag (Vitarine) | aluminum hydroxide | |
| | gel | n.s. | |

| | | | |
|---|---|---|---|
| 35. | Magnesia and Alumina Oral (Philips Roxane) | aluminum oxide | — |
| | suspension | 24 mg/ml | 55 |
| 36. | Mylanta (Stuart) | aluminum hydroxide | |
| | tablet | 200 mg | 58 |
| | suspension | 40 mg/ml | 58 |
| 37. | Mylanta II (Stuart) | aluminum hydroxide | |
| | tablet | 400 mg | 116 |
| | suspension | 80 mg/ml | 116 |
| 38. | Noralac (No. American) | bismuth aluminate | |
| | tablet | 300 mg | 55 |
| 39. | Nutrajel (Cenci) | aluminum hydroxide | |
| | suspension | 60 mg/ml | 87 |
| 40. | Pama (No. American) | aluminum hydroxide | |
| | tablet | 260 mg | 75 |
| 41. | Riopan (Ayerst) | magaldrate | |
| | tablet | 400 mg | 51 |
| | suspension | 80 mg/ml | 51 |
| 42. | Riopan Plus (Ayerst) | magaldrate | |
| | tablet | 480 mg | 61 |
| | suspension | 80 mg/ml | 51 |
| 43. | Robalate (Robins) | dihydroxyaluminum sodium carbonate | |
| | tablet | 500 mg | 94 |
| 44. | Rolaids(Warner-Lambert) | dihydroxyaluminum sodium carbonate | |
| | tablets | 334 mg | 63 |

| | | | |
|---|---|---|---|
| 45. | Silain-Gel (Robins) | aluminum hydroxide | |
| | tablet | 282 mg | 83 |
| | suspension | 56 mg/ml | 83 |
| 46. | Syntrogel (Block) | aluminum hydroxide | |
| | tablet | 38% | — |
| 47. | Trimagel (Columbia Medical) | aluminum hydroxide | |
| | tablet | 250 mg | 72 |
| 48. | Trisogel (Lilly) | aluminum hydroxide | |
| | capsule | 100 mg | 29 |
| | suspension | 30 mg/ml | 43 |
| 49. | WinGel (Winthrop) | aluminum hydroxide | |
| | tablet | 180 mg | 52 |
| | suspension | 36 mg/ml | 52 |

n.s.—not specified·

For those of you who use buffered aspirin to avoid gastric upset, which is sometimes caused by the use of regular aspirin, you should be aware that you may be consuming between 200 and 1,000 milligrams of aluminum per day, especially if the dosage taken is from 3 to 9 grams of buffered aspirin daily. Two extra-strength buffered aspirins, the dosage recommended every four hours, equals one gram. So should you take the recommended dose three times in any given day, you would have ingested three grams of buffered aspirin. Alternatives do exist, such as aspirin buffered with calcium carbonate and time-released aspirin, which does not contain any added aluminum.

For a detailed analysis of such analgesics, or *buffered aspirins* that contain aluminum, table 5 will be useful.

Table 6 discloses the aluminum content of some antidiarrheal drugs.

**Table 5:** Nonprescription Internal Analgesics (Buffered Aspirins) Containing Aluminum

| | Brand name (manufacturer) | aluminum salt (concentration) | aluminum content per tablet (mg) |
|---|---|---|---|
| 1. | Arthritis Pain Formula (Whitehall) | aluminum hydroxide n.s. | — |
| 2. | Arthritis Strength Bufferin (Bristol-Myers) | aluminum glycinate 73 mg | 15 |
| 3. | Ascriptin (Rorer) | aluminum hydroxide 75 mg | 22 |
| 4. | Ascriptin A/D (Rorer) | aluminum hydroxide 150 mg | 44 |
| 5. | B-A (O'Neal, Jones & Feldman) | aluminum hydroxide 100 mg | 29 |
| 6. | Pabrin (Dorsey) | aluminum hydroxide 100 mg | 29 |
| 7. | Bufferin (Bristol-Myers) | aluminum glycinate 49 mg | 10 |
| 8. | Cama (Dorsey) | aluminum hydroxide 150 mg | 44 |
| 9. | Cope (Glenbrook) | aluminum hydroxide 25 mg | 7.2 |
| 10. | Vanquish Caplet (Glenbrook) | aluminum hydroxide 25 mg | 7.2 |

n.s.—not specified

**Table 6:** NonPrescription Antidiarrheal Drugs that Contain Aluminum

| | Brand Name (manufacturer) | Aluminum salt (content/tablet or ml suspension) |
|---|---|---|
| 1. | Amogel (No. Amer.) | kaolin, 120 mg |
| 2. | Bisilad (Central) | kaolin, 370 mg/ml |
| 3. | Diabismul (O'Neal, Jones & Feldman) | kaolin, 170 mg/ml |
| 4. | Donnagel-PG (Robins) | kaolin, 200 mg/ml |
| 5. | Donnagel (Robins) | kaolin, 200 mg/ml |
| 6. | Kaolin Pectin Suspension (Philips Roxane) | kaolin, 190 mg/ml |
| 7. | Kaopectate (Upjohn) | kaolin, 190 mg/ml |
| 8. | Kaopectate Concentrate (Upjohn) | kaolin, 290 mg/ml |
| 9. | Pabisol with Paregoric | aluminum magnesium silicate, 8.83 mg/ml |
| 10. | Parepectolin (Rorer) | kaolin, 180 mg/ml |
| 11. | Pargel (Parke-Davis) | kaolin, 200 mg/ml |
| 12. | Pektamalt (Warren-Teed) | kaolin, 217 mg/ml |
| 13. | Quintess (Lilly) | attapulgite, 100 mg/ml |
| 14. | Rheaban (Pfizer) | attapulgite, 600 mg/tablet, 140 mg/ml suspension |

Before leaving this category of aluminum absorption, we should point out that some hemorrhoidal medications and antiperspirants, which are applied topically, may also contain aluminum. However, neither category contributes any substantial amount of this metal through absorption.

## Occupational Sources of Aluminum

Some industries and occupations create higher levels of aluminum in the working environment than average, and these should be taken into consideration when assessing your overall intake of aluminum. Occupational exposures include:

Aluminum welding;
Manufacture of aluminum abrasives,
products, and alloys;
Manufacture of aluminum metal powders;
Manufacture of paper, glass, porcelain, explosives,
textiles (waterproofing), and synthetic leather;
Manufacture and use of pyrotechnical devices;
Production of alumina and alum from bauxite ore.

## Eliminating Aluminum in the Kitchen

It is in the kitchen that we can make significant inroads in our quest to eliminate this metal from our lives.

Let's begin with the obvious. First, use aluminum foil very sparsely and never to wrap highly acidic or highly alkaline foods. For example, if aluminum foil is used to preserve leftover pizza for just a few days, you may notice small holes in the foil. This is because the acidic nature of the food (the tomato sauce in the pizza) has caused the absorption of aluminum out of the foil into the food product. Using aluminum pots to brew and reheat acidic drinks such as coffee may add significant quantities of aluminum to your overall intake. By using an aluminum pot to cook a food such as tomatoes, the resultant absorption can increase the amount of aluminum taken in by your body up to 2 to 4 milligrams per serving.

By using cookware made of aluminum, you may increase the amount of aluminum taken in each day by between 9 and 17 percent.

A new source of aluminum in our diet is the aluminum-coated waxed container, utilized especially for orange and pineapple juices. Both juices will absorb this suspect metal from the inside of the container; exact amounts are not yet determined. Common sense would lead us to purchase juices in non-aluminum-coated containers.

Beer stored in aluminum cans absorbs small quantities of the metal, according to a German study by F. Ullman. The longer the beer is stored, the higher is the amount absorbed. For this reason I suggest choosing beer in bottles.

Some products are secured with an aluminum seal over the top of the container. Such use seems to be all right as long as the seal does not contact the food.

In table 7, under the heading "Aluminum Content of Tomatoes Cooked in Aluminum or Porcelained-Iron Pot," you will see that aluminum cookware contributes significantly to the amounts of aluminum in our diet, particularly when compared to a porcelainized iron pot. You will note that the use of aluminum pots can increase the aluminum content of tomatoes, a typically acidic food, by between 2 to 4 milligrams per serving.

While many more studies are needed before we can say with any certainty the effects of using aluminum cookware to prepare various foods, it does seem advisable that Alzheimer's patients, and those of us who want to reduce the risk of succumbing to Alzheimer's, should make a careful effort to reduce aluminum in the kitchen and elsewhere in our lives.

**Table 7:** Aluminum Content of Tomatoes Cooked in Aluminum or Porcelained-Iron Pot

| Sample | Dry weight (g/ml) | mg Al/ 100 g[10] | mg Al/60 ml serving (4) |
|---|---|---|---|
| Before cooking | 0.059 | 1.31 | 0.046 |
| P-I[11] pot, 2 hrs | 0.118 | 1.13 | 0.080 |
| Al pot, 2 hrs | 0.102 | 31.7 | 1.94 |
| P-I pot, cooked 2 hrs, stored overnight | 0.130 | 1.00 | 0.079 |
| Al pot, cooked 2 hrs, stored overnight | 0.123 | 52.9 | 3.89 |

## Is It Really Necessary to Change My Cookware?

The question of the safety of aluminum was raised back in the 1920s when it first appeared in the form of cooking pots. It has remained largely submerged in the health food literature. However, on July 17, 1980, Dr. Steven Levick, M.D., of the Yale University School of Medicine, wrote a letter to the *New England Journal of Medicine* in which he hypothesized a connection between the use of aluminum cookware and Alzheimer's disease.

Dr. Levick wrote, that, as a "financially strapped medical student," he had used inexpensive aluminum pans and pots. After using them for two years he noticed, "corrosive pitting and whitish powdery deposits around the pots." Connecting this finding with the known observation that higher-than-normal levels of aluminum are found in the brain tissue of deceased

10 Al assays were done in the laboratory of John Crispin Smith, Trace Metals Unit, Kettering Laboratory, University of Cincinnati Medical Center, Cincinnati, Ohio.

11 P-I: porcelained-iron pot.

victims of Alzheimer's disease, Dr. Levick raised the issue of the potential toxicity of aluminum in Alzheimer's disease. Needless to say, he never used his inexpensive aluminum pots again.

It is generally known that highly acidic foods and beverages attract and absorb aluminum from cookware. Be aware, however, that highly *alkaline* foods also absorb this toxic metal. Alkaline foods corrode pots more rapidly even than acidic foods! These foods attract aluminum, and an aluminum hydroxide gel is formed. In the stomach these alkaline compounds are converted into acidic aluminum compounds.

So, the more time highly acidic or highly alkaline foods and beverages remain in aluminum cookware, the more aluminum will enter the food. When using aluminum, be concerned about sauerkraut, citrus juices, and tomato sauce. In the chart below note that garlic, onions, spinach, swiss chard, tomatoes, and eggplant—all commonly associated with Italian food—are alkaline and likely to attract aluminum from cookware. Such highly acidic items as coffee are also chemically "attractive" to aluminum.

Instead of calculating which foods are acidic or alkaline you should simply invest in a new set of pots. When eating in restaurants, be advised; cheap aluminum cookware is the norm.

## The Acid-Alkaline Chart

| Acid | Highly Acid | Neutral |
|---|---|---|
| Beans (kidney, navy, white, garbanzo) | Alcohol | OILS: |
| Beef | Artichoke | Avocado |
| Blueberries | Barley | Olive |
| Brussels sprouts | Bread | Sesame |

| Acid | Highly Acid | Neutral |
|---|---|---|
| Cashews | Buckwheat | Coconut |
| Coconut, dried | Caffeine | Soy |
| Cranberries | Corn, dry yellow | Sunflower |
| Egg yolk | Custards | Safflower |
| Filberts | Drugs | Cottonseed |
| Fish | Flours (all) | Almond |
| Fruit (dried, sulfured, canned, sugared, jams, jellies) | Ginger, preserved | Linseed |
| Gelatin | Honey | |
| Goat, meat and dairy | Lentils, dry | FATS: |
| Grapes, sweet | Maté | Butter |
| Milk products, pasteurized | Millet | Cream |
| Mushrooms | Oatmeal | Margarine |
| Mutton | Peanuts | Animal fat |
| Pecans | Potato, sweet | Lard |
| Plums, Damson | Rice (all) | |
| Pork | Rye grain | |
| Poultry | Sorghum | |
| Sorghum grain | Soy, bread and noodles | |
| Water chestnuts | Spaghetti products | |
| | Squash, except winter | |
| | Sugar, cane and raw | |
| | Tobacco | |
| | Walnuts, English | |
| | Wheat grain | |

| **Alkaline** | **High Alkaline** | **Highly Alkaline** |
|---|---|---|
| Agar | Almonds | Beans, dried lima, string |
| Alfalfa | Avocado | Bean sprouts |
| Apple and cider | Banana, speckled only | Currants |
| Apricot, fresh | Beans, fresh lima | Dandelion greens |
| Artichokes, globe | Beet | Dates |
| Asparagus | Blackberries | Figs, especially black |
| Bamboo shoots | Carrot | Prunes |
| Beans, snap | Chives | Swiss chard |
| Berries, most | Cranberries | |
| Bok choy | Endive | |
| Broccoli | Grapes, sour | |
| Cabbage (red, white, savoy, Chinese) | Kale | |
| Cantaloupe | Peach, dried | |
| Cauliflower | Persimmon | |
| Celery | Plum | |
| Cherries | Pomegranate | |
| Chestnuts | Raspberries | |
| Chicory | Spinach | |
| Coconut, fresh meat and milk | | |
| Coffee substitutes | | |
| Collards | | |
| Corn, fresh sweet | | |
| Daikon | | |
| Eggplant | | |
| Escarole | | |
| Garlic | | |
| Ginger, dry | | |

| Alkaline | High Alkaline | Highly Alkaline |
|---|---|---|
| Gooseberries | | |
| Guava | | |
| Horseradish, fresh raw | | |
| Kelp | | |
| Kohlrabi | | |
| Leek | | |
| Lemon and peel | | |
| Lettuce | | |
| Lime | | |
| Loganberries | | |
| Mango | | |
| Melons | | |
| Milk (raw, whey, yogurt, acidophilus) | | |
| Nectarine | | |
| Okra | | |
| Olives, sun-dried | | |
| Onion | | |
| Orange | | |
| Papaya | | |
| Parsley | | |
| Parsnip | | |
| Peach, fresh | | |
| Pear, fresh | | |
| Peas | | |
| Pepper, green and red | | |
| Pineapple, ripe | | |
| Potato, except sweet | | |
| Prickly pear | | |

| Alkaline | High Alkaline | Highly Alkaline |
|---|---|---|
| Pumpkin | | |
| Quince | | |
| Radishes | | |
| Rhubarb | | |
| Sapodilla | | |
| Sauerkraut, lemon | | |
| Squash, winter | | |
| Tamari | | |
| Tangerine | | |
| Teas (clover, sage, mint, strawberry, alfalfa) | | |
| Tomato | | |
| Turnip | | |
| Watercress | | |
| Yeast | | |

Developed by Anabolic Foods, Irvine, California.

What kinds of cooking pots are available other than aluminum?

There are many affordable alternatives. These include stainless steel, glass, well-glazed pottery, tin-lined copper, and iron cookware. Of course, non-stick pans are also perfectly acceptable.

When checking your cookware, please look carefully at older, decorated metal cookware, including their lids. Before the early 1970s, some foreign manufacturers decorated some of this type of cookware with brightly colored cadmium-containing enamels. This cadmium, especially in older cookware, can migrate from the cookware into the food being prepared.

While china crockery and earthenware are ancient in their use for cooking and storage, it is important for you to inspect modern versions of this cookware. More recent technology has determined that some of the pottery production methods used can be hazardous to your health. By inspection, be certain that the glazes that were used on them are properly applied and fired.

You can test this by rubbing vigorously with a white cloth and detergent. No color from the applied decoration or color tint should be removed by the cloth. If there are fine, multiple hairline cracks over the surface of your pottery cookware (what is commonly called "crazing"), the pottery is either very old, in which case it should not be used, or the glaze has been incorrectly fired and will not seal in the metallic-based color tint of the pottery or the decoration. Such cookware should not be used for food preparation, serving, or storage.

Most ceramic or pottery cookware must be fired several times at a high temperature to seal permanently the decorative colors under the glaze. Some Italian and Mexican pottery and cookware that has been improperly glazed may permit acidic or salty foods to react with the potentially hazardous lead and cadmium-containing paints used in the decoration, thereby presenting a hazard and possible toxicity.

My secretary is from an English family in the heart of the Staffordshire potteries. She told me the following story about the hazards of lead.

Her cousin, a hand painter of figurines for a major British pottery (where they used lead-containing paint), suffered several miscarriages. A smart doctor decided to test her blood for an elevated lead level. The level was dangerously high from inhaling the paint fumes. It took over a year (out of work and away from painting) before the lead level receded sufficiently for her to conceive and finally carry a healthy child to term.

Finally, the amateur potter may not be completely aware of the proper methods of mixing the ceramic substance used and of the proper firing time and temperature needed to make their products suitable for use with food. Such cookware may be better used for decorative purposes instead of being used for cooking and storing food.

I recently enjoyed a meal in my favorite, much frequented, Italian restaurant in New York City. As a token of his appreciation for my patronage, the owner presented me with the beautifully decorated, Italian wine pitcher that was used to serve my wine that night. Upon arriving home with my gift, I followed my practice of inspecting all highly decorated pottery to determine their safety. I noticed many hairline cracks throughout the interior of this wine pitcher, including cracks at the pouring lip.

While gazing at this pitcher, I wondered if any of the paint used in the decoration contained lead and, if so, how much of this lead may have leached into the wine I drank during my meal that night.

This brought to mind an anecdote presented by social scientist S. Colum Gilfillan, as mentioned in Dr. Michael Lesser's book *Nutrition and Vitamin Therapy*. He hypothesized that the Roman Empire collapsed largely owing to the fact that the Romans used crockery and wine goblets that contained large amounts of lead, and water to wealthy homes was carried in lead pipes. Thus, lead leached into the food, water, and wine of the ancient Romans and slowly poisoned them.

Symptoms of lead poisoning include lethargy, confusion, a loss of memory, and an inability to concentrate. If this hypothesis is correct and ancient Rome fell, in part, due to a large ingestion of lead, let's not repeat the mistake and see Western civilization succumb to Alzheimer's disease, brought about, in part, by aluminum poisoning!

## How Do We Determine If We Have Excess Aluminum in Our Systems?

If you are now concerned that you may have ingested an excess amount of aluminum from your diet, or from your cookware, and would like to determine what that level is, a simple method is available to you.

While hair analysis is often *not* accurate for most minerals, it fortunately is extremely accurate in telling us what our levels of the *heavy metals* are, such as mercury, lead, and cadmium. Hair analysis is also a good indicator of excessive *aluminum* exposure.

While the increase in hair aluminum may not correlate directly with the amount of hair produced, nor with the amount of aluminum ingested over a period of time, hair analysis should be useful for indicating any increase of aluminum in your system over what would be considered "normal."

One of the most accurate methods of testing is known as "flameless atomic absorption analysis of acid-digested hair samples." Such a test can be ordered through your physician or health practitioner. A full report on the effectiveness of hair analysis, entitled "Hair as an Indicator of Excessive Aluminum Exposure," appears in *Clinical Chemistry* (volume 28, number 4, pages 662 to 665, 1982) and should convince even the most skeptical physician of the value of this laboratory test.

Let us now look at some current treatments for Alzheimer's disease and then go on to the heart and soul of our risk-reduction program: chelation and nutrition.

# 5

# CURRENT THERAPIES[12]

In chapter six, we will see how some controversial treatment methods (chelation and nutrition) are slowly being introduced in the treatment and prevention of Alzheimer's disease. In this chapter we will take a look at the more conventional treatments (which, in some cases, are quite effective) and learn how they can interact with other suggestions in this book.

Most of the current conventional therapies involve medication and drugs. While these drugs do not prevent the illness or eliminate it, they do slow progress and give comfort to victims; so they should be understood by those affected by Alzheimer's. The categories of drugs most often used are:

1. nootropics (piracetam)
2. stimulants (amphetamines)
3. vasodilating agents (hydergine, papaverine, and others)

12 This chapter is based, in part, on the excellent discussion in *A Guide to Alzheimer's Disease* by Barry Reisberg, M.D., Free Press, 1981. References to studies mentioned here can be found on pages 140–45 of Dr. Reisberg's book.

4. neuropeptides (vasopressin)
5. procaine solution (G-H3)
6. neurotransmitters or their precursors

Each one's action within the body and interactions with the metabolic and nervous systems will be briefly explained.

## Nootropics (Piracetam)

The first medication on our list is among the most promising for treatment of dementias. The group name for these medications, "nootropics," means simply "mind" and "toward," and it is hoped that these drugs will improve the memory in patients suffering from Alzheimer's and other diseases affecting memory loss.

Among this group of nootropics is a drug known as piracetam. In testing on animal subjects, the drug seemed to improve learning ability and also appeared to protect the animals from losing their memory in conditions of low oxygen (such as appears to be the case with some victims of dementia). Further testing on these animals showed that the drug had increased the electrical activity in that part of the brain where impulses are carried between the cerebral hemispheres. From this testing, the researchers believed that the drug piracetam actually increased the speed with which information is usually passed from one hemisphere of the brain to the other.

It has been reported in studies on human subjects that a group of students given piracetam prior to an exam did considerably better than did a group of students taking the same exam who were given a placebo instead of piracetam.

Further testing has been done on aged adults, some exhibiting no symptoms of memory impairment and others with a moderate amount of age-related memory dysfunction. In both cases, piracetam appeared to improve behavior and thinking ability. These tests suggest that piracetam improves memory and retention of input regardless of whether any dysfunction exists.

Unlike other medications that affect the mind, piracetam does not relieve pain, induce sleep, or tranquilize the patient. Heart rate, blood pressure, and cerebral blood flow ail remain constant during piracetam medication treatment. The one and only thing that piracetam seems to accomplish is the increase in energy stored by the brain, thus enhancing memory retention. Or, in the case of memory dysfunction, restoring and repairing the damage.

When virtually every medication on the market today has some side effect, one of the most amazing aspects of piracetam is that it seems to have absolutely none on either animal or human subjects! Due to the newness of the drug, this is said with great caution. But all testing thus far does seem to indicate that this drug will play an increasing role in treating Alzheimer's disease.

Although this drug is now in use in many areas of the world, it is presently being used only experimentally in the United States. Once investigations are completed, we will be able to ascertain the usefulness of using piracetam to treat senility and the early stages of dementias such as Alzheimer's disease.

Another drug that may be classified as a nootropic, and one that is about to be approved for medical usage in the United States, is called Vinpocetine. The drug was discovered in the early 1970s in Hungary and is now being used in Mexico, Japan, and Eastern Bloc countries.

This chemical has been shown to enhance memory and improve disturbances of daily living in several important studies, without serious side effects. The drug holds great promise and will no doubt be welcomed in the treatment of Alzheimer's disease.

While many solid studies attest to the benefits of Vinpocetine, the most recent contains a complete list of earlier studies and is cited in the bibliography (see Peruzza, 1986).

## Stimulants (Amphetamines)

This is a group of medications known more commonly to the drug culture of today simply as "uppers." The two most common amphetamines are prescribed under the trade name Dexedrine© which is dextroamphetamine sulfate, and Benzedrine© which is amphetamine sulfate.

These medications are supposed to sharpen your attention and lift your mood. In reality, the reverse effect has often been observed. An hour after receiving the medication, many patients experience feelings of fatigue and sleepiness. When these sleepy patients were tested, measured electrical activity in the brain was reduced, demonstrating a loss of alertness, the opposite of the result desired from the medication. So where in some cases the term "upper" is applicable for the first hour, a "downer" follows with an undesirable depression.

Other medications in this group, such as pentylenetetrazol, sold under the trade name of Metrazol©, and methylphenidate, sold under the trade name Ritalin©, have been equally disappointing in the treatment of dementias such as Alzheimer's disease. Unfortunately, methylphenidate is prescribed by doctors all too frequently.

One out of every seven prescriptions written for a psychostimulant in the United States is for the treatment of symptoms related to senility. Yet a recent review by the Food and Drug Administration concluded that amphetamines, when used for treating senility, are lacking in effectiveness.

### Vasodilating Agents (Hydergine, Papaverine, and Others)

The former, widely held theory that senility was a result of the progressive narrowing of the blood vessels in the brain, caused by the accumulation of arteriosclerotic deposits, brought about the introduction of vasodilator treatments. This treatment is used to expand the narrowed blood vessels.

Today, medical consensus is that Alzheimer's disease is the major cause of senile dementia and that senility due to vascular involvement, such as multi-infarct dementia, accounts for the greater percentage of the balance of all other senilities. The difference is that unlike Alzheimer's disease, multi-infarct dementia is aligned with the condition of arteriosclerosis, which is a narrowing and blocking by an accumulation of calcium and fatty deposits of the arteries throughout the body.

Knowing that a lack of oxygen to the brain can, even for a relatively short period of time, cause permanent brain damage, it was not surprising for researchers to discover that the body had a built-in natural protective device.

Through experimentation, it was discovered that carbon dioxide is a natural dilator (widening mechanism) of the cerebral blood vessels, thus allowing more oxygen-rich blood to flow through them and reach the brain in times of need. Should testing of patients show a higher-than-average buildup of carbon dioxide in their body tissues, it would indicate to the doctor that they are lacking a supply of sufficient oxygen, possibly due to narrowing of their arteries. Thus the use of a vasodilator such as carbon dioxide in the treatment of dementias.

Surprisingly, Alzheimer's victims show a slightly better response to vasodilator treatment than do multi-infarct dementias. Possibly, this is related to the different possible causes of the two dementias.

Multi-infarct dementia patients have blood vessels that have become stiff from atherosclerotic deposits, making them inflexible and not so easily dilated.

As Alzheimer's disease appears to be caused by factors other than narrowed or blocked arteries, Alzheimer's patients' arteries are able to respond to vasodilating treatment, thus allowing more oxygen-rich blood to reach brain cells.

"Dihydroergotoxine" (a carbon dioxide vasodilator), is the vasodilator most widely studied and used in the treatment of senility. It is composed of a fungus that grows on rye and other cereal grains. A study of institutionalized Medicaid patients in California revealed that dihydroergotoxine was number two on the list of total drug expenditures in that state.

There have been several clinical studies using dihydroergotoxine in the treatment of elderly victims suffering from various degrees of dementia, with some small measure of positive results. A degree of continued minor improvement was evident during one three-month experiment. The longest period of study in the United States using dihydroergotoxine was only of six-months duration.

In Europe, a fifteen-month study of nursing home residents was conducted using dosages of 4.5 milligrams of dihydroergotoxine (a slightly higher dosage than is usually recommended) and compared to a placebo group within the same facility.

After six months, neither the patients receiving dihydroergotoxine nor the placebo showed any evidence of improved general intelligence. However, studies of blood flow showed a decline in the placebo patients while the dihydroergotoxine-treated patients did show improvement in the blood flow to the brain. Alzheimer's victims who received dihydroergotoxine treatment in this study also showed improvement in the brain's electrical activity, in comparison to the Alzheimer's victims who received the placebo.

At the end of the fifteen-month period, studies of general intelligence and blood flow showed a further decline in patients that received the placebo while the patients receiving dihydroergotoxine exhibited a slight improvement in intelligence testing and cerebral blood flow.

Thus far, the evidence of dihydroergotoxine's positive effect on Alzheimer's patients and dementias in general is encouraging. Perhaps future studies, extending over a longer period of time (for example, two or more years) will provide us with more information concerning proper dosage and long-term effects.

Papaverine (marketed as Pavabid©) is another chemical substance used to improve brain blood flow. This substance is found in opium; however, it does not have any of the narcotic influences one might expect.

It has been found effective in relaxing the involuntary muscles and increasing blood flow to the brain. Papaverine has been tested with several good scientific protocols, showing some value in the treatment of an assortment of different forms of senility.

Similar to dihydroergotoxine, studies of patients treated with papaverine from one and a half to two years have shown the greatest positive response.

Following a two-year study of patients who received papaverine, definite improvement was recorded in the brain's electrical activity in 50 percent of the patients while the other 50 percent showed no improvement. However, of the patients who had received a placebo in place of papaverine, two-thirds showed a deterioration of their brain activity.

When comparing the treatment of senile dementia patients using papaverine and the treatment using dihydroergotoxine, short-term clinical studies conclude that dihydroergotoxine is the better choice.

There are other vasodilator drugs available today, such as cyclandelate (Cyclospasmol©) and isoxsuprine (Vasodilan©). At the present time, evidence supporting the effectiveness of dihydroergotoxine and papaverine is definitely the most convincing.

## Neuropeptides (Vasopressin)

Neuropeptides have created quite a bit of excitement in recent years and may prove useful in the treatment of senility and memory impairment. Neuropeptides consist of amino acids, the basic structure from which proteins are formed. Amino acids in short chains are commonly called peptides. Peptides have been found to affect the nervous system, hence the name, neuropeptides.

The ongoing discovery of neuropeptides and their role in monitoring and controlling the functions of the body is so prolific that current information is outdated shortly after it is printed. Interest in this class of drugs in the scientific community came about after it was discovered that removal of an animal's pituitary gland decreased its ability to learn.

There are several groups of neuropeptides, of which one group seems to control the pain perception received by the brain, such as the message to pull a finger away from a flame. Certain other peptides act as hormones and the conveyers of messages and instructions between body cells, tissues, and organs. These peptides are known as transmitters.

To understand why neuropeptides are such an important medication in the treatment of disorders affecting the mind, we have to first understand the major role of our pituitary gland.

Often referred to as the "master gland," the pituitary synthesizes hormones that influence many other important glands, such as the thyroid, sex glands, and the adrenals. It is also the site of the production of hormones that directly influence numerous functions of the body.

In laboratory testing, it has been observed that individual hormones such as melanocyte-stimulating hormone (MSH), adrenocorticotropic (ATCH), and vasopressin, can reverse the loss of learning ability produced by the removal of the animal's entire pituitary gland. Through further testing it was ascertained that these hormones acted directly with the brain, independently of the adrenal glands, and appeared to improve learning ability.

Unfortunately, human experiments with ACTH or MSH have not yet had very encouraging results. Vasopressin on the other hand is producing quite promising results and may become one of the first neuropeptides used in the treatment of senility and dementias such as Alzheimer's disease.

This possibility was further demonstrated in laboratory testing. One experiment employed a strain of rats with a congenital defect, the inability to produce vasopressin, which renders them incapable of retaining the memory required to perform learned tasks.

Scientists discovered that by injecting vasopressin into the rats, it was possible to improve their learning ability. And even more encouraging, the injection also enabled the rats to remember responses previously taught that they had forgotten.

## Procaine Solution (G-H3)

This form of treatment, developed by the Romanian physician Dr. Ana Aslan, is Gerovital-H3 (G-H3) and commonly referred to as "Romanian procaine" after its inventor and its major active ingredient, procaine. The solution actually consists of 2 percent procaine hydrochloride and is more commonly known as Novocain, a local anesthetic.

The chemical messengers (neurotransmitters) with which nerve cells communicate must be quickly broken down to allow new messages to be sent. This breakdown is achieved by the use of enzymes, the major one of which is monoamine oxidase (MAO). Procaine's benefit in treating depression and other disorders affecting the mind is its ability to lessen or inhibit the action of the enzyme MAO. As an "MAO inhibitor," procaine or G-H3 acts to *increase* the amount of neurotransmitters. Thus, an extra, or now adequate, quantity of these chemical messengers is made available, possibly explaining their action.

MAO inhibitors are also used in psychiatry on younger patients for the treatment of severe depressions that may also be due to a depletion or insufficient quantities of neurotransmitter chemicals in the brain.

As MAO activity increases with aging, an inhibition of its action with a medication such as G-H3 can alleviate certain types of depression related to aging.

Obviously, G-H3's use for improving memory loss in the aged would be limited to those patients whose memory loss was due to depression or mood-related imbalance. Senile dementias and Alzheimer's disease patients would receive little, if any benefit by treatment with any MAO inhibitors.

## Neurotransmitter Precursors or Agonists

The evidence implicating the decreased activity of the enzyme CAT, which is necessary for the production of acetylcholine, in the body of Alzheimer's patients is overwhelming. It has been found that the more severe the case of Alzheimer's disease, the greater is the decrease in the enzyme level of CAT in the patient's body.

Any agent that could increase the quantity of acetylcholine in the brain would be of great benefit in the treatment of Alzheimer's disease and other senile dementias. A few such treatments had been experimented with, such as choline salts that can be ingested orally, with little or no success. Drs. Little and Levy, of King College Hospital, London, did, however, achieve success with high dosages of lecithin.

The greatest source of choline for the body and, in particular, for the brain is achieved through diet. Lecithin contains phosphatidyl choline (which is found in our cellular membranes) and is a natural source of choline. Many foods contain lecithin, such as egg yolks, brewer's yeast, soybeans, fish, beef liver, peanuts, wheat germ, and whole grains, and are readily available. A supplement would be in order for those of us interested in reducing risk of Alzheimer's disease.

A study conducted by Etienne and coworkers, based on dietary choline supplementation in the form of lecithin for Alzheimer's patients has been reported in *Lancet* (Etienne, P., et al., "Clinical Effects of Choline in Alzheimer's Disease," 1:508-09, 1978). In this published report, it was suggested that three out of seven Alzheimer's patients treated with lecithin showed improvement. This path of treatment is of great interest to many medical researchers and scientists and should shortly be passed on to Alzheimer's patients.

While lecithin supplementation is very promising, it is *not* pharmacologic, depending to a great extent on diet. For this reason we devote a large portion of the next chapter to this promising "natural" treatment for Alzheimer's disease.

Other chemical approaches stimulating the response to acetylcholine by nerves in Alzheimer's disease are being conducted. A chemical has been developed that inhibits an enzyme that destroys acetylcholine when it is released. Physostigmine, the chemical used, has been shown to effectively raise the quantity of the acetylcholine neurotransmitter.

Experiments with physostigmine do show a positive indication that improvement in the mental function of Alzheimer's and other dementia patients can be achieved. However, at the moment, the correct dosage has not been ascertained. As too little or too much physostigmine is not beneficial, more research will have to be accomplished before this chemical can be ascertained as being therapeutic for a dementia treatment.

Further experimentation is being conducted using lecithin and physostigmine in conjunction with each other. Thus far, the preliminary results appear promising, according to L. J. Thal and coworkers at the Albert Einstein Medical Center in New York.

The experimental drug THA, recently lauded for its beneficial effects in a small group of Alzheimer's patients, is good news for a nutrition-oriented person. What this drug does is help maintain levels of acetylcholine, the critically important nerve messenger. The scientists who reported their initial success in the study group of Alzheimer's patients openly acknowledged the several previous studies that showed similar beneficial effects from the administration of choline, the nutrient. (See *The New England Journal of Medicine*, November 13, 1986, page 1244). "The administration of more than 8 grams of choline chloride or its equivalent for more than three weeks has produced moderate improvement in subjects with early Alzheimer's disease."

In concluding our review of the current conventional treatments for Alzheimer's disease and other dementias, our most optimistic choice is to use a dietary treatment with lecithin. Of all the other treatments reviewed, while they may bring a degree of relief and/or an easing of symptoms, possibly even slowing the progress of the disease, none of them is a cure for Alzheimer's disease.

In the last chapter, we will discuss nutrition and list the different foods and supplements that will work naturally toward preventing and possibly alleviating the severity of

Alzheimer's disease. These dietary "interventions" offer us the most *positive* steps we can take in our risk-reduction program. In the next chapter we will see which *negative* steps we can follow to eliminate aluminum, a possible culprit in causing or exacerbating Alzheimer's disease.

# 6

# REMOVING *YOUR* EXCESS ALUMINUM

In the high mountains of Ecuador in South America, there is a village, nestled in a valley, where some of the longest-lived people on earth reside. The village is called Vilcabamba. Here in this valley, approximately nine or ten people out of the total population of eight hundred have ages well over one hundred. In the United States of America, with almost 250 million people by comparison, there are scarcely a few dozen people over the age of one hundred!

From an epidemiologist's point of view, this valley has been of immense interest. Because the birthdates of the people of Vilcabamba can be verified by baptismal records, this village has been studied in great detail by a team from Harvard University.

When meeting the people of this peaceful Eden, your gaze is immediately drawn to the alert brightness of their eyes, the youthful smiles on their faces, and you ask yourself, "Could these people really have lived this long on this earth?" Some of the natives of Vilcabamba are over 130 years old!

In this valley there is no retirement age; the elderly people all work. There is no rocking chair to complete our image of elderly people. Slowly, methodically, they all go about their various daily chores, walking up the hill to the field to tend to their crops, gently hoeing between the plantlings. Back down the hill they come and on to chopping a few logs. This they may do several times a day. In between, they may pause to draw water from the well or sit busily plaiting a rope or spinning the cotton for their clothing. These people are all active, alive, and functioning happily.

Of course, there are complex social factors that may help explain the greater longevity enjoyed by these blessed people.

Sexuality is treated as naturally as it could be anywhere on earth. People experience their needs and practice them well into the end of their days. There is no such thing as a concept of a "dirty old man" or a "dirty old woman" in this valley. People understand their needs and act on them peacefully and in accord with the laws of nature.

When interviewers posed the question to these vibrant, elderly people, "Why have you lived so long and enjoyed such good health?" they gave various reasons as their answers.

One delightful woman of 112, with eyes twinkling, showing radiance and vivacity, attributes her longevity to the good water in the river that they drink from and from the sweet smell of the beautiful flowers and trees that surround them. Another native of the village, well into his hundreds, claims that his longevity and strength is due to the bears he has killed and eaten every few years or so.

Others gave different reasons, but seldom did we find that diet was the chief reason given. The shocking truth is that many of these people smoke anywhere from forty to sixty cigarettes each day. Of course the tobacco is not store-bought. It is locally grown, without pesticides, without chemical fertilizers, and smoked without undergoing the numerous processes used to treat our tobacco. The cigarettes are not wrapped in the commercial paper that we use, but wrapped in their own leaves, or even in toilet paper when they can get it! Also, these people generally drink anywhere from two to four cups of rum a day. However, the rum is unrefined, made from locally grown sugar cane.

On the dietary level though, I am happy to report that the people of this valley of longevity do eat a largely vegetarian diet that consists chiefly of grains. Their protein intake is only about one ounce per day. Their fat intake is very modest, and the rest of their diet consists of grains, corn, yucca, beans, and potatoes supplemented with oranges, bananas, and other fruits. Their total caloric intake is only about 1,700 calories per day, which is quite low even compared to the average intake in other developing countries.

Incidentally, senile dementia or Alzheimer's-like states are completely unknown in this community.

## Natural Chelators

Is there something we can learn from these long-lived people of the valley of Vilacabamba that may help us protect ourselves from Alzheimer's disease?

As we said earlier, aluminum is a ubiquitous metal found virtually everywhere on earth. It is the third most abundant element in the crust of the earth, making up 8 percent of the total. It does not occur naturally in the elemental form, but is found in compounds, such as oxides and silicates. Aluminum is also widely distributed in many plants. The roots act as reservoirs for this metal, with the seeds and blossoms also containing some.

The people in the Ecuadorian valley are no doubt exposed to aluminum, from their food and their water, as well as from the earthen floors upon which they sleep. And yet, if the aluminum enters their bodies, why does it not wind up in their brain, bound to their neurons?

In the healthy adult, there are numerous physiological mechanisms in operation that prevent most aluminum from being absorbed and distributed to the brain. It is only when a person has impaired kidney function, some other abnormal physiology, or when they are super-saturated with aluminum from their environment (sources such as food, water, medicine, deodorants, etc.) that some of this metal is deposited where it does not belong in the brain and neurons, thus bringing about neurotoxicity.

Not being exposed to the excess, commercial sources of aluminum, the people of this Ecuadorian village are thus able to rid themselves of this toxic metal through their diet and lifestyle, which act as natural chelators.

## What Is Chelation?

In its original Greek form, this word referred to the prehensile claws of crabs and lobsters. Medically, the term means an agent with the ability to "grab" another compound and, it is hoped, remove it.

Progressive physicians, albeit few in number, are utilizing a technique in which a proteinlike material is introduced that binds with or "chelates" calcium and other metals in the bloodstream. This complex is later excreted from the body through the urinary system.

In the case of Alzheimer's disease, chelating with an amino acid called EDTA may remove aluminum from brain tissue as well as restoring elasticity to cerebral arteries, thereby increasing brain blood flow. Another chelating agent, desferrioxamine, is being utilized experimentally by Dr. McLachlan's research group at the University of Toronto with preliminary promising results. Additionally, this chelating agent is now being employed to remove aluminum from the brain cells of people from Guam suffering from an Alzheimer's-like syndrome. This research is being conducted by a group from the U.S. National Institutes of Health (NIH). The results of the Toronto research have been submitted to the *Journal of Pharmacology and Experimental Therapeutics* and are pending publication. According to T. P. A. Kruck, Dr. McLachlan's associate and the principal author of this new study, aluminum is definitely removed by chelation. Due to the advanced age of his subjects, clinical data were poor. A new study will be tried on younger victims of Alzheimer's disease (mean age seventy-two), with more promising clinical results expected. The title of the first-mentioned unpublished study is "Removal of Brain Aluminum by Ion-specific Chelation in Alzheimer's Disease."

Let's imagine for a moment that our blood vessels are a water supply system, or the pipes in our home. After many, many years of use, you know that the pipes in your home become corroded and obstructed by mineral deposits (from the water) causing rust and deterioration, necessitating their repair or replacement. If there would be some way to clean the interior of these pipes, they could be used for many more years to come.

As it turns out, we have internal mechanisms for cleansing our blood vessels. It is simply through moving our muscles and keeping oxygen-rich blood flowing through them. By moving our muscles, the accumulated wastes are carried away instead of being deposited on the interior of the arteries.

If we are physically active, thus stimulating and ensuring that we enjoy a good flow of oxygen in our bloodstream and the proper elimination of the waste products from our systems, the formation of plaque and the occlusion of arteries to our brain and other vital organs is retarded. This is why aerobic exercise, in conjunction with a fiber-rich diet, is a natural method of chelating toxic metals from our body.

While there is some controversy as to just *how* chelation achieves results, there is little doubt that it does so. The Harvard Medical School-trained physician Elmer M. Cranton, M.D., in his excellent book *Bypassing Bypass*, states, "There is no evidence that chelation therapy reduces plaque size in humans. On the other hand, there is a wealth of evidence that the symptoms of reduced blood flow improve in more than 75 percent of patients treated." We will see in the case studies discussed later in this chapter that improving blood flow to the brain can greatly reduce memory loss and other symptoms associated with Alzheimer's disease.

As we stated at the beginning of this chapter, the people of the Ecuadorian valley are physically active each and every day of their lives, until the very end. They do not retire. Their diet consists of a high amount of unrefined carbohydrates, very small quantities of animal protein, and very small quantities of fat. This type of high complex carbohydrate diet, combined with aerobic exercise, is the key to longevity. The lesson we can learn from the people of Vilacabamba is that by following an ancient pattern of activity, and a more ancient dietary pattern, we can naturally maintain arterial elasticity and a youthful blood flow.

But as we know, the process of chelation is a very slow one. An early demonstration used to explain how chelation works from diet alone was illustrated by an actual experiment that can be done at home. For this experiment you follow a simple Asian recipe for spare ribs. If you put a group of small bones in a dish and soak them in vinegar for several days, you would notice how the bones become thinner and softer. It was thought this happened because vinegar, which is a weak acid, would have chelated calcium out of the bones.

Current thinking rejects this model, preferring instead the theory that chelation removes harmful free-radical compounds. In either case, a lifetime of eating natural chelating foods and aerobic exercise should help prevent the accumulation of aluminum and other harmful metals in our system. Not only will we protect ourselves from excess accumulation of aluminum, but excess lead, mercury, cadmium, arsenic, and even iron.

## Foods that Chelate Aluminum

Fortunately, there are *foods* that naturally chelate aluminum, lead (a highly toxic metal), and other undesirable minerals. The amino acids cysteine and methionine are known as sulfhydryl-containing because they are especially rich in sulfur. When sulfur is combined with hydrogen, they form such sulfhydryl groups, which are very effective in removing poisons and toxins.

Foods that provide us with aluminum-removing sulfhydryl groups are readily available and may explain, in part, why senility of the Alzheimer's type is unknown among the long-lived people of Ecuador.

Foods such as onions, garlic, chives, red pepper, and egg yolks contain relatively large amounts of sulfur compounds and are all natural chelators of toxic metals.

Have you noticed how asparagus changes the odor of your urine, often soon after the vegetable is eaten? This is due to the sulfur-bearing compounds contained in this desirable vegetable.

Another excellent dietary source of sulfhydryl groups are such foods as pea beans, limas, pintos, kidneys, soybeans and other legumes, all of which remove aluminum and are advised for your risk-reduction program. Sesame, pumpkin, and sunflower seeds as well as English walnuts all contain ample methionine and should be eaten regularly as snack foods.

In addition to the above chelating foods, in chapter seven we will discuss the vitamins, minerals, and amino acids that are specifically recommended for their natural chelating properties.

## Has Chelation Helped with Actual Alzheimer's Victims?

A key proponent of chelation treatment is Dr. Richard Casdorph, M.D., Ph.D., formerly Assistant Clinical Professor of Medicine at the University of California Medical School, Irvine, California.

Dr. Casdorph was trained in cardiology at the Mayo Clinic and, in addition, received his Ph.D. degree in Medicine from the University of Minnesota. He taught at UCLA

Medical School and was Chief of Medicine at the Long Beach Community Hospital.

Recently, Dr. Casdorph looked at the effects of EDTA[13] chelation therapy in brain disorders, including Alzheimer's disease, and reported a significant increase in the flow of blood to the cerebrums in all but one of fifteen patients treated. This improvement in cerebral blood flow generally took approximately twenty chelation treatments. And, while he stated that all fifteen patients showed clinical improvement, one improved without any increased blood flow to the brain. He ascribes this clinical improvement to the fact that EDTA chelates and removes aluminum.

One of Dr. Casdorph's patients was a 51-year-old white female who had been clinically diagnosed as schizophrenic. She had exhibited symptoms of depression and isolation and a pattern of sleeping for unusually long periods of time.

Following admission to the hospital for an unrelated condition, a brain-blood-flow study was performed. The results showed gross abnormalities. Chelation therapy was explained to the patient and her husband, after which they elected to begin EDTA treatment. While treatment was going on, the patient showed visible signs of improvement, becoming more outgoing, and she even, for the first time since her illness began, drove herself to the doctor's office.

After thirteen infusions of EDTA, a follow-up brain-blood-flow study showed great improvement. At the completion of

13 Critics of chelation therapy rightly state that EDTA *too* broadly removes all minerals, including critically important trace metals. For this reason the chelating agent desferrioxamine, which is ion-specific to aluminum, is now being utilized experimentally.

twenty infusions of EDTA, a further brain-blood-flow study revealed marked improvement.

Another patient of Dr. Casdorph's was a 72-year-old white female. This patient was in a vegetative state as a result of long-standing hypertension (high blood pressure). Clinical tests had shown evidence of cerebral atrophy (withering of the brain), which explained her deteriorated mental state. This patient did not even recognize her husband, to whom she had been married for fifty years. She was experiencing hallucinations and delusions, forcing her husband to consider institutional care for her.

Following neurological evaluation and testing, the patient was started on chelation therapy. At the completion of only six infusions, all signs of mental deterioration had diminished. The patient was now rational and completely oriented to her surroundings and family, and even her vision had improved. There was no longer a need for nursing home care.

After twenty infusions of EDTA, much to Dr. Casdorph's dismay, the repeated brain-blood-flow study showed no further significant improvement. Undiscouraged, six more infusions of EDTA were performed, and the next brain-blood-flow study showed a significantly improved condition of this patient.

With restricted cerebral blood flow (due to contracted cerebral blood vessels) and long-standing hypertension (high blood pressure), a 62-year-old female is our third example of the results of chelation therapy. Brain-blood-flow studies on this woman indicated gross abnormalities. Twenty infusions of EDTA were given, after which the brain-blood-flow studies showed a return to nearly normal, much improving this patient clinically.

The first male patient in our examples is a 57-year-old white male. This man had suffered a cerebrovascular accident (commonly called a stroke), which had left him with right-sided hemiparesis (partial paralysis affecting muscular motion but not sensation). Brain-blood-flow studies again were performed, showing gross abnormalities. Marked improvement was achieved following twenty infusions of EDTA.

Another patient, a 66-year-old white female, had multiple problems, which included long-standing diabetes mellitus, requiring insulin treatment. She was obese and suffered from multiple complications related to her diabetes, including diabetic retinopathy (a major cause of blindness), nephropathy (kidney disease), neuropathy, with atherosclerosis obliterans (thickening and hardening of the inner walls of an artery), and other serious problems.

Again, brain-blood-flow studies initially showed abnormalities that were greatly improved following twenty infusions of EDTA.

Dr. Casdorph also reports treating a 76-year-old white female, clinically diagnosed as having Alzheimer's disease. Tests were performed and confirmed the evidence of cerebral atrophy. Prior to treatment, brain-blood-flow studies showed marked evidence of abnormality. After twenty infusions of EDTA a significant improvement in her mental functioning was achieved, and a further brain-blood-flow study demonstrated marked improvement.

Our final case study is a 92-year-old white male with confirmed evidence of cerebral atrophy. Brain-blood-flow studies demonstrated abnormalities, but after six infusions of EDTA, he showed a little improvement. Following the final brain-blood-flow study, after twenty EDTA infusions, significant improvement was achieved, but some abnormalities did still remain.

## Conditions Requiring Precaution with Chelation or "Some Potential Side Effects"

Chelation is not a miracle cure and should *not* be used by everyone! Several side effects have been reported to the AAMP Scientific Advisory Committee: loss of appetite, thirst, chills, back pain, abdominal cramps, muscle cramps, skin eruptions, anemia, tiredness, and an overall unwell feeling. At the completion of treatment, however, all of these side effects disappear rapidly. They can be alleviated during treatment by the reduction of EDTA chelation dosage.

To elaborate further on specific side effects and the corrective measures that have been used to alleviate such symptoms, the following is a detailed list of conditions needing special precaution for anyone interested in considering chelation.

### Congestive Heart Failure

Patients with congestive heart failure (inadequate heart function, shortness of breath, and swollen ankles) require special handling during EDTA chelation therapy. The medication (digitalis) used to treat congestive heart failure is decreased in its effectiveness during EDTA treatment. The congestive heart failure patient is also often unable to cope with the excess of fluid from the intravenous feeding and/or the sodium content. Thus, his condition could become aggravated during treatment. The treating physician must lower the sodium intravenous vehicle for congestive heart failure patients by using dextrose or fructose.

## Diabetes

Diabetic patients who are maintained by protamine zinc insulin may become hypoglycemic with a resultant insulin shock reaction, as the EDTA therapy could cause this long-acting type of insulin to be released too quickly. The initial response to such a reaction is to get sugar into the patient immediately and then switch to a different type of insulin.

On the more positive side, diabetics being treated with other types of insulin are benefited by EDTA chelation therapy as the therapy will usually cause a gradual decrease in their insulin requirements.

## Hypoglycemia

Prior to chelation treatment, it is recommended that high calcium-containing foods, such as dairy products, and most sugars, including overripe bananas, should be avoided. Instead, to avoid the possibility of a hypoglycemic reaction, with its unsettling symptoms of irritability, depression, and sleepiness, a diet of sufficient unrefined complex carbohydrates is recommended. To further avoid this side effect, eating nourishing fruit, such as a fresh banana, during infusion will help to lessen a hypoglycemic reaction. Monitoring of the blood pressure during treatment is also done by your physician to identify any signs of an adverse reaction.

## Postural Hypotension

As EDTA chelation therapy lowers your blood pressure during infusion, it can cause postural hypotension. While benefitting patients with hypertension (high blood pressure), it may lower the blood pressure of patients with normal levels to the point that dizziness may be experienced upon standing up too quickly. This side effect is easily remedied by raising to an upright or standing position more slowly, thus giving your blood pressure a chance to elevate itself.

## Hyperthyroidism

EDTA chelation therapy has been known to alter the metabolism rate. The resultant reaction suffered by the patient is a slowed metabolic rate causing sluggishness, fatigue, and weight gain. This condition is easily corrected by supplementing with trace minerals that include iodine.

On the more positive side, EDTA chelation therapy can have a reverse effect. A patient already suffering from an under-functioning thyroid (hypothyroidism) may very well find his condition alleviated and, not uncommonly, returned to normal functioning.

## Thrombophlebitis

If a patient is known to have blood-clot problems, heparin will probably be added to the EDTA solution. Occasionally, thrombophlebitis is a side effect of chelation therapy. Should this occur, moist heat applied to the affected area and adequate supplies of natural antioxidant nutrients, such as vitamin C, vitamin E, and selenium, will ease and protect against this condition.

However, it has been reported that some vitamin E supplements actually have no vitamin E activity in them (indicating a low or nonexistent level of action of the compound) and may contain instead rancid oil, which could actually cause thrombophlebitis. An orthomolecular physician would be your best source of advice as to which brands of vitamin E are reliable and readily available to you.

## Fatigue and Weakness

As chelation therapy may deplete the levels of trace minerals including magnesium, potassium, or zinc ions in the body cells, extreme fatigue and weakness may be experienced. To counteract this reaction, eating foods that are high in potassium, such as bananas, is the usual successful remedy. In addition, these trace minerals must be taken as supplements to maintain the delicate electrolyte balance.

## Discomfort

Some people are more sensitive than others and feel uncomfortable even when a solution is correctly entering a vein. To ease any sensation of discomfort or local irritation, magnesium chloride, magnesium sulfate, or procaine is sometimes added to the intravenous solution.

## Diarrhea

Diarrhea is another possible side effect of chelation therapy. It is usually overcome with standard antidiarrheal treatment.

However, since many antidiarrheal drugs contain aluminum, only those *without* aluminum should be utilized. See your pharmacist for a list of ingredients.

## Vomiting and/or Nausea

Occasionally, a few chelation therapy patients may experience nausea and possibly vomiting. Extra-high doses of pyridoxine (vitamin B-6) have prevented such symptoms. A possible causative effect of nausea and vomiting is that chelation therapy may pull this nutrient, pyridoxine, out of the body.

## Headaches

Eating certain foods during infusion, such as bananas, nuts, and seeds, especially during the first hour of treatment, have been effective toward preventing headaches, another possible side effect of chelation therapy. Aspirin or other analgesics may be safely used to relieve the pain of headaches. Following this regimen, physicians administering chelation treatment report that, in most cases, this side effect is completely eliminated.

## Fever

In some cases, a fever is experienced by patients receiving chelation therapy, the reason for which is unclear. It could be an allergic response to one or more of the several ingredients contained in the solution, or simply that the patient is coming down with a cold or flu virus.

## Skin Inflammation

Vitamin-mineral supplements taken as a preventive measure can ensure adequate levels of zinc and pyridoxine. Lack of these essential nutrients during chelation therapy can produce an exfoliative dermatitis such as shedding or peeling of the superficial skin layers.

## Neurological Effects

Another possible side effect is of a neurological nature, namely, pins and needles, numbness, and a sensation of tingling around the mouth area. This is a temporary sensation caused by the infusion entering the vein too fast and is easily remedied by slowing the rate of the infusion solution into the vein.

## Aches and Pains

The "overchelation" syndrome is another possible side effect. It is demonstrated by flulike symptoms, complete with aching joints. This usually occurs in a few patients receiving chelation therapy two or three times a week. The problem is solved by either decreasing the number of chelation therapy treatments to once a week and/or lowering the dose of ingredients used in the infusions or decreasing the rate with which the infusion enters the vein.

As you can see, the side effects, although numerous, are mostly minor ones, or are easily remedied. It is suggested that you discuss these side effects with your physician before making a decision to enter into EDTA chelation therapy.

## Who Should Not Take Chelation Treatments?

There are several types of patients who should probably not elect chelation therapy. In some cases contraindication may be overruled, based on the benefit likely to be received and despite the danger posed by an existing contraindicating ailment. However, your physician should not entertain the idea of chelation therapy *without* first establishing your current physical well being by extensive examination and clinical diagnostic procedures and testing. Testing is also important as a tool for documenting your improvement during the course of EDTA chelation treatment.

Here are some contraindications to chelation therapy and the exceptions that may be considered.

### Cranial Lesions and Tumors

Brain tumors and lesions are often a contraindication to chelation therapy. Chelation therapy may remove calcium from the body and in so doing could bring about a convulsion in patients suffering from such conditions. Several factors pertaining to the need and the potential benefit, weighed against any possible risk, would determine if such a patient were a candidate for chelation therapy.

### Liver Disease

Most liver diseases contraindicate chelation therapy. These include chronic or toxic hepatitis, cancer, and most other serious liver problems. Ironically, chelation therapy has been proven helpful to patients with chronic cirrhosis of the liver.

## Nutritional Deficiencies

Vitamin or mineral deficiencies are a contraindication to chelation therapy. Extensive biochemical evaluation of the patient's nutritional deficits must be done before chelation therapy is started. Once such deficiencies are identified, the patient's nutritional health can be restored permitting initiation of chelation therapy.

## Tuberculosis, Inactive

The potential risk of chelation therapy to patients with inactive tuberculosis is that the tuberculosis could become active as a result of the therapy, the reason being that old, calcified tubercular lesions could, during chelation therapy, be stripped of the calcified covering. This could allow the bacillus organism to become reactivated, thus putting the patient into an active tuberculosis state again.

With the development of new medications that have proven very effective against tuberculosis, this risk could be lessened. This allows both active and inactive tuberculosis patients to be treated with chelation therapy, provided that careful monitoring is performed during therapy. The benefits of therapy versus the risks involved would have to be carefully weighed before any decision was made.

## Advanced Kidney Disease

Chelation therapy requires a relatively healthy kidney to dispose of the chelated toxic waste removed from the body during EDTA treatment.

Only in very extreme cases, such as a longer life expectancy with chelation therapy, would a physician entertain the possibility of this type of treatment in a patient with kidney disease. It would then be performed only with extreme caution. In general, advanced kidney disease patients are not candidates for chelation therapy.

### Moderate Kidney Disease

Chelation therapy can be performed on patients suffering from moderate kidney disease provided extreme care and monitoring is exercised. However, the therapy would not be performed as frequently or in as high doses as it would be normally. The dosage would be at least one half or less of the usually prescribed dose until such time as the patient's kidney disease showed signs of improvement.

Moderate kidney dysfunction patients can receive chelation therapy, again, provided it is handled with caution. The dosage and frequency *would* be lessened and careful monitoring performed throughout. Taking sauna baths during therapy is also thought to be helpful as sweat can help eliminate toxins and metals from the body, thus assisting the kidneys and enhancing the effects of chelation therapy.

## To Chelate or Not to Chelate?

The best way to conclude our evaluation of chelation therapy is to offer you a "second opinion." Again, we turn to Elmer Cranton, who, in addition to having earned his M.D. degree from Harvard Medical School, is board certified as a specialist by both the American Board of Chelation Therapy and by the

American Board of Family Practice. He also utilized EDTA chelation therapy "for approximately ten years, with marked and lasting benefit in 75 to 95 percent of hundreds of patients treated. Observed benefits have correlated with the total number of treatments. No harm has come to any of these patients as a result of EDTA therapy."

And what does this medical expert have to say about Dr. Casdorph's findings?

"Dr. Casdorph's second study, which measures brain-blood flow, contains even more convincing data to prove that EDTA chelation therapy results in a very significant improvement in circulation to the brain. The probability that these results could have been due to random chance are less than five in ten thousand. That study was duplicated and confirmed independently by other researchers using a different technology." (E. Cranton, *Bypassing Bypass*, pp. 107-8.)

Whether or not you elect chelation for yourself or a family member WILL be dependent on many factors that you must evaluate.

In either case, by eating those naturally chelating foods discussed earlier in this chapter, you will be doing much in the way of reducing the risk of accumulating aluminum in your brain cells and other organs. And, as pointed out earlier, "aluminum should be considered toxic to both brain and bone, at least until compelling evidence proves otherwise." (G. H. Mayor and co-workers, Department of Medicine, Nephrology Division, College of Human Medicine, Michigan State University, East Lansing, Michigan.)

We will now turn to other specific *nutritional* components of our risk-reduction program.

# 7

# IMPROVING NUTRITION FOR A HEALTHY BRAIN

While it is too early to say for certain where, or if indeed there is, a single "trigger" that sets off the Alzheimer's disease process, we do know that the nutritional program outlined below will help achieve a positive outcome. The high levels of aluminum found in the diseased brain cells of Alzheimer's patients can likely be avoided and reduced. In this chapter we will focus on dietary methods.

Before looking at a program of prevention based, in part, on nutrition, let's turn back to the circumstantial evidence given us by the Chamorro natives of Guam in the Western Pacific (as well as in parts of New Guinea and Japan).

As you may remember, these island people suffered from an unusually high incidence of a type of dementia in combination with Parkinson's disease called amyotrophic lateral sclerosis, or ALS. These patients all had high levels of aluminum, iron, and calcium in their diseased brains. And, as was noted before, abnormally high levels of aluminum and low calcium and magnesium levels occur in their drinking water and garden soils. ALS has largely disappeared in Guam with the introduction of diets richer in calcium- and magnesium-bearing foods.

That a lifetime of inadequate calcium and magnesium intake can lead to a *deposition* of calcium in brain cells is readily explained. According to D. C. Gajdusek, the Nobel Prize-winning researcher now at the National Institutes of Health who has studied ALS for over twenty years, long-term deficiencies of these minerals may alter parathyroid function. Thus, "Alterations in mineral metabolism ... could render dangerous otherwise harmless trace mineral excesses, making them chronically toxic to the motor neuron. This could occur because of increased gastrointestinal absorption and decreased deposition in bone and decreased renal excretion with resulting increased deposition ... in the soft tissues, including the brain." (Dr. Gajdusek in Chen and Yase, 1984; "Amyotrophic Lateral Sclerosis in Asia and Oceania.")

Thus, it may be possible that the hormonal mechanism that is designed to regulate calcium levels in the body picks up and begins to use aluminum as a substitute. Several experiments with animals have shown that when there is a shortage of calcium in the diet, more aluminum will be absorbed from foods and taken up by the brain. Whatever the mechanism, there is a significant similarity between ALS and Alzheimer's disease: neurofibrillary tangles, in large quantities, form in the brains of victims of both disorders! The neurofibrillary tangles in both diseases have been linked to a buildup of aluminum in brain cells.

Professor James Edwardson, of the Medical Research Council, Newcastle, England, believes, at this early stage, that elderly people may, in fact, develop senile plaques owing to a similar deficiency in calcium. This can begin quite early in life or simply be a process of the later years. So called "secondary hyperparathyroidism" is traced to a lack of calcium and magnesium, which encourages a deposit of other metal ions in the brain. While we have focused on the aluminum deposited in the brain cells of Alzheimer's patients, bromine, mercury, and silicon are sometimes present as well. These other metals are likely deposited due to the same irregularity in the calcium balance.

Elderly people have several factors playing at once that tend to upset their calcium balance, both in their blood and tissues. These range from diet through genetic and environmental factors, as well as the possibilities described earlier, such as a virus that might upset the mineral balance in the nervous system, leading to the formation of aluminosilicates (aluminum combined with silicon).

When the stomach fluids become highly acidic, any aluminum present in the diet or drugs will collect and be transported into the bloodstream. Elderly people who tend to have highly acidic stomach fluids may use a lot of antacids. This puts them in a prime state for absorbing the aluminum that is part of their antacid tablets, as well as the aluminum found in cooking pots, deodorants, processed cheeses, and other sources we have mentioned. We have known for years that even mildly elevated levels of aluminum can influence memory disturbances in adults as well as hyperactivity and learning disorders in children. It does not matter to Alzheimer's patients whether these elevated levels of brain aluminum are a cause or a result of the disease. What we want to do is remove this toxic metal if it is present, or prevent it from being deposited in the first place.

As I mentioned earlier, there are many published scientific papers that indicate that aluminum increases the permeability of the barrier between the blood and the brain and that this permits harmful substances to enter the brain.

Professor R. J. Boegman, Department of Pharmacology and Toxicology, Queens University, Kingston, Ontario, Canada, an early worker in this field, suggests that when aluminum is deposited in the gray matter of the brain, it will inhibit nerve transport, increase the breakdown of various neurotransmitters, and stimulate the production of harmful proteins. The consequences of aluminum deposits can include seizures, a decreased ability to learn, an impaired motor coordination, memory loss, and even psychotic reactions.

## Aluminum Plus Silicon: The Core of This Molecular Bombshell

At the center of Alzheimer's disease are the senile plaques described earlier in this book. These are spherical regions of brain nerve terminals in decay; they surround a core material called amyloid. This amyloid is composed of a type of protein, found only in these senile plaques, combined with large amounts of aluminum and silicon.

These *aluminosilicates* were discovered by Professors J. M. Candy, J. A. Edwardson and coworkers, of Newcastle General Hospital, England. The form in which these two elements were found was not previously noted to have occurred in the nervous system. This unusual chemical combination can expand and may also act as a catalyst to speed the breakdown of surrounding, normal proteins. This may explain why aluminum damages brain cells.

## Malnutrition and Malabsorption May Be the Key

"Observable pathology does not necessarily account for a disorder," as has been suggested by those skeptical of "The Aluminum Connection." However, whether aluminosilicates are only a *consequence* of, or actually *cause*, the disease is not of prime importance. To *prevent* their occurrence is our concern.

Before looking at specific nutrient deficiencies that are associated with the buildup of aluminosilicates, we should look at the hypothetical basis upon which our discussion is based. Using the idea that *malnutrition* may be the key element, or the key process underlying this disease, we should keep in mind that psychological or sociological causes by themselves do not necessarily have to be excluded. As we know, depression can also induce malnutrition, as can loneliness in the elderly, who simply stop eating.

It is also important to remember before proceeding that this concept of malnutrition and Alzheimer's disease may also be related to *malabsorption*. Simply improving the feeding of patients does not always guarantee that the nutrients will be absorbed. And further, in some patients we can only obtain a normal serum albumin level by *massive* protein feeding, not by the feeding of normal amounts.

Malabsorption is generally recognized by clinicians by two signs, diarrhea or constipation. And yet the absence of diarrhea and the presence of constipation does not rule out malabsorption. All of these observations have been reported in the literature and recorded in an interesting paper by F. Abalan from Bordeaux, France, as reported in *Medical Hypotheses* (volume 15; pp. 385 to 393, 1984).

In addition to malabsorption, there is a decreased metabolism of blood sugar and oxygen in the brain of Alzheimer's patients. Strangely, all of these indicators of malnutrition can be brought about by a protein-calorie malnutrition syndrome, which is generally exhibited by a body weight less than 90 percent of ideal weight and a low blood-protein level (under 35 grams per liter). It is also important to note that a person of normal weight, or even an obese person, may still be suffering from protein-calorie malnutrition because edema, or the slow mobilization of fat, can actually hide tissue loss.

## The Essential Fats

Often overlooked in discussions of nutrition and Alzheimer's disease are the lipids, or fats. Remember this: certain fatty acids are essential. They cannot be produced by the body but must be taken in from the diet. The brain in particular is highly sensitive and must have a sufficient supply of these essential fatty acids, or cofactors, including vitamin B-6, vitamin C, and zinc.

The essential fatty acid is known as linoleic acid; in order for our biochemistry to proceed, this essential lipid must be desaturated or broken down. The ability to do so decreases with age and is almost entirely lost, because of functional liver damage, in alcoholics, who then become emaciated, as we know, and quite often demented.

Another group of lipids that are critical, if not essential, is known as the omega-3 fatty acids. These are found in abundance in cold-water fish such as salmon, mackerel, herring, albacore tuna, whitefish, anchovy, bass, and Atlantic cod.

Table 8 provides a list of fish and their omega-3 content. All are beneficial and should be eaten in abundance. In addition to supplying us with lipids, which nourish our brain, we will also reduce our risk of heart attacks, according to numerous studies with Greenland's Eskimos.

**Table 8:** The Omega-3 Content of Fish

| **Fish** | **Omega-3 Fatty Acids (Grams per 3 ½ oz.)** |
|---|---|
| Mackerel, Atlantic | 2.6 |
| Herring | 1.7 |
| Salmon, Chinook | 1.5 |
| Tuna, Albacore | 1.5 |
| Whitefish, Lake | 1.5 |
| Anchovy | 1.4 |
| Bass, Striped | 0.8 |
| Oyster, Pacific | 0.6 |
| Trout, Rainbow | 0.6 |
| Halibut, Pacific | 0.5 |
| Shrimp, Northern | 0.5 |
| Crab, Alaska King | 0.3 |
| Cod, Atlantic | 0.3 |
| Swordfish | 0.2 |
| Lobster, Northern | 0.2 |
| Red Snapper | 0.2 |
| Scallops | 0.2 |
| Flounder, Yellowtail | 0.2 |
| Haddock | 0.2 |
| Sole, European | 0.1 |

## Other Missing Nutrients

In addition to low levels of essential fatty acids, there are other nutrient deficiencies common in Alzheimer's patients. These include deficiencies of the essential amino acids phenylalanine and tryptophan; vitamins B-1, riboflavin, B-6, B-12, choline, pantothenic acid, and vitamin C; several minerals, particularly calcium; and trace elements. These nutrients and their food sources are discussed later in this chapter.

## Malnutrition: A Common Denominator

As we have seen earlier, many hypotheses exist to explain Alzheimer's disease. These include genetic causes, bacteria, viruses, toxic compounds (such as aluminum), biochemical abnormalities, and a poorly functioning immune system. None of these have been proven, and none of them *alone* can explain the full range of the biological, anatomical, and clinical picture as described in this disease. Yet it may be that *malnutrition* is the underlying issue, both because this condition permits aluminum to deposit in the brain and prevents the utilization of choline and other critical nutrients.

A leader in the theory of malnutrition being a possible cause of Alzheimer's disease is Dr. Francois Abalan, of Centre Hospitalier Charles-Perrens, Bordeaux, France. At a recent symposium, Dr. Abalan proposed that both malabsorption of nutrients and inadequate intake of critical nutrients may contribute to Alzheimer's disease. He further offered the concept that "Nutritional treatment would seem to improve moderate forms" of Alzheimer's disease.

The following malnutrition prototype is derived from Dr. Abalan's work. He is presently conducting a detailed trial of nutritional treatment of Alzheimer's disease. And, based on his initial results, we can soon expect an encouraging report.

If we look at Alzheimer's patients, we will almost always see the following conditions present. Patients are generally emaciated, particularly toward the end of the disease. There are almost always urinary tract infections, a terminal type of bronchopneumonia, a low triceps skin fold (at the rear of the upper arm), as well as low blood levels of certain nutrients. In the chart below, the nutrients often deficient in Alzheimer's patients appear on the left while good food sources appear on the right.

| DEFICIENT NUTRIENT | FOODS TO EAT |
|---|---|
| Albumin (simple proteins) | Milk; egg whites |
| Iron (which diminishes as the number of senile plaques increases) | Liver (beef or lamb); beef; baked beans; apricots; prunes; soybeans; lima beans; spinach |
| Folic Acid | Liver; yeast; leafy vegetables (lettuce, broccoli); asparagus; fresh oranges; nuts; legumes; whole wheat |
| Tryptophane (an amino acid) | Milk; complex carbohydrate foods |
| Vitamin B-12 | Liver and other organ meats; raw clams; oysters; sardines; herring |
| Niacin (called by Dr. Abalan vitamin PP, meaning "Pellagra Preventative") | Brewer's yeast; fish; liver; chicken; whole grains; nuts; legumes |

## Why Nutrients Do Not Always Work

Skeptics have sometimes argued that choline, lecithin, tyrosine, and tryptophan have not always worked with Alzheimer's patients. Well, there may be a very simple explanation for this. These nutrients are considered *precursors* and must be converted into other compounds before they can be utilized by our bodies and brains. If we lack the necessary enzymes and other nutritional "assistants" that occur in the forms of vitamins, minerals, and trace elements, these precursors are totally useless. Although little is being done in the United States, many psychiatric hospitals in France are beginning to use such factors in the form of pancreatic enzymes, corticosteroids, and adrenocorticotropic hormones, as well as vitamins, without realizing that these constitute a form of nutritional therapy. These nutrients actually ameliorate the disease, according to Dr. Abalan.

Let us now look at specific vitamins, trace elements, minerals, and essential fatty acids that may be useful in preventing and treating this disease.

## Essential Nutrients for Reducing Risk

In the following detailed look at the vitamins, minerals, lipids, and amino acids, please bear in mind that several of them are highly critical in preventing and treating this illness, both theoretically and practically. The vitamins we want to look at are vitamins A, B-l, B-6, B-12, folic acid, choline, and vitamin C. In addition, we want to avoid *vitamin D*, because the metabolites of this vitamin increase absorption of aluminum.

As far as the minerals go, we want to pay particular attention to calcium, magnesium, and zinc. As for the lipids (or fats), we want to pay attention to linoleic acid (that is an essential fatty acid), lecithin, and the omega-3 fatty acids. Under the amino acids, we will look at tyrosine and tryptophane. Finally, we want to pay attention to the relative acidity of our stomachs. Aluminum compounds that we may take in from foods, antacids, and other sources are far more soluble in acidic solutions. Therefore, we want to make certain that our stomachs are not unbalanced too far to the acid side.

In the following discussion, several other vitamins, minerals, and amino acids will also be discussed. However, as pointed out, the vitamins, minerals, amino acids, and lipids named above are necessary to metabolize choline and lecithin, which may explain why some experiments using these substances have been equivocal in their results. That is, the patients did not also receive the other required nutritional "assistants" in the forms of vitamins, minerals, and trace elements. Finally, we will look at how to select a multi-vitamin and mineral formula that will help us get all of the above nutrients plus others beneficial to our overall health.

## The Vitamins

### Vitamin A

Vitamin A is often associated with maintenance of proper vision and prevention of night blindness, but it does much more than that. A powerful antioxidant and free-radical[14] deac-

14 Free radicals are formed during metabolic processes or contributed by pollutants, toxicants, certain drugs, and food processes. These highly reactive molecules may attach to other incomplete molecules and form carcinogenic or otherwise destructive compounds.

tivator, this valuable vitamin helps to protect against the potential damage from released free radicals. It helps to stabilize the cellular membranes. It is also an important stimulant to the immune system and protects the thymus, the gland associated with the immune system.

Because it promotes the normal development of epithelial tissue (the membranes in our body) vitamin A protects against cancer of the skin, lung, and other epithelial tissues, where nearly half of all human cancers begin. A major, recent study (Menkes, et al., *New England Journal of Medicine*, November 13, 1986, pages 1250-54) confirmed the value of vitamin A in protecting us against lung cancer. While this vitamin had been touted in the "health-food" literature for its antitumor benefits for years, only recently have major studies been undertaken to test the validity of this "grass-roots" science. As this study has shown, certain nutrients can protect us against cancer. Hopefully, future studies will explore the potential benefits of nutrients against Alzheimer's disease.

Vitamin A is also needed in the manufacture of the antistress hormones of the adrenal cortex and is used up under stressful conditions, including the stress incurred with Alzheimer's disease. Signs of vitamin A deficiency include insomnia, fatigue, depression, nerve pains in the extremities, and sore eyes, symptoms that are common to patients in nursing homes.

Because it is soluble in fat rather than water, vitamin A can be toxic in excessive doses since it can accumulate in the fatty tissues of the body. It is important, therefore, to take vitamin A with other antioxidants, such as vitamins E and C and the mineral selenium, since these will help protect vitamin A from oxidation, thereby reducing the requirement for vitamin A itself.

The safest form in which to take this vitamin is beta-carotene, as found in vegetables. This is less toxic than other forms of vitamin A.

Good plant sources of this vitamin are the green and yellow vegetables. Remember, the depth of the yellow or green color is a rough guide to the amount of vitamin A in the vegetable. Carrots, apricots, sweet potatoes, squash, cantaloupe, pumpkin, and other deeply colored fruits and vegetables are the preferred food sources of this important vitamin.

As a quick frame of reference, one 3-ounce carrot contains about 11,000 IUs of vitamin A (as B carotene). While the recommended daily allowance (RDA) is very low (about 5,000 IUs for an adult), I recommend an intake of between 25,000 to 50,000 IUs per day, from all sources (foods and vitamin pills). The toxicity symptoms begin over 75,000 IUs in an adult.

## Vitamin B Complex

The B vitamins are grouped together because they tend to occur in the same foods and they do similar work in the body. They should be taken in combination as B complex because some of the B vitamins help the body to use others.

In general, the B vitamins are known for their ability to help deal with stress. For the minimally oxygen-starved brain of the Alzheimer's patient, they are an essential factor in dealing with depression and fatigue, maintaining energy, and calming the nerves. One B vitamin, choline, is so important in treating the nervous system that it will be dealt with separately.

Other members of the vitamin B complex, described below, also serve functions that are of special help in brain function.

Pantothenic acid (another B vitamin) is an important anti-stress vitamin. It is also involved in the production of acetylcholine in the brain and nervous system and in energy metabolism.

Inositol (also part of the B complex) may be helpful in combating insomnia. Its mild, antianxiety effect often makes it a useful, natural alternative to mild prescription tranquilizers.

Vitamin B-l, or thiamin, is involved in the conversion of blood sugar to caloric energy in the body. During stressful periods it can give a boost to your energy level. Thiamin can be depleted by poor diet and by overuse of caffeine and tobacco. The need for thiamin is also increased by the use of antidepressants.

Thiamin deficiency, or beriberi, is known to produce psychiatric and neurological symptoms, which might be mistaken for senile changes in an elderly person.

A form of brain disease known as Wernicke-Korsakoff syndrome results from a partial destruction of the brain owing to the lack of thiamin; this condition is most commonly found in chronic alcoholics but has been diagnosed in nonalcoholics as well. The symptoms are similar to those of senile dementia, with memory problems being the first to appear. The use of thiamin has been shown to reverse the clouded consciousness of Wernicke-Korsakoff syndrome in clinical studies.

Since thiamin deficiency, or an increased need for thiamin, is the main cause of Wernicke-Korsakoff syndrome, Abram Hoffer suggests that thiamin be added to alcoholic beverages as a way of preventing the disease. A divided dosage of 250 milligrams a day is recommended. The consumption of large quantities of refined sugar can also produce a thiamin deficiency state, since thiamin is essential to sugar metabolism.

This vitamin is *essential* to our risk-reduction program and must be taken in through foods and/or supplements each day. Thiamin is not as easy to get from foods as it once was. Processing foods destroys this sensitive vitamin as does cooking. Raw nuts, legumes, and whole grains are good sources, as are green, leafy vegetables. Wheat germ added to dishes is a convenient means of supplementing this and other vitamins of the B complex.

If you like meat and are not prone to elevated blood-cholesterol levels, organ meats and pork flesh are abundant sources of thiamin. We should remember that sugar and fats, which make up a high percentage of processed foods and supply over 35 percent of our calories, give us no thiamin or other B vitamins. Finally, excessive use of tea, alcohol, and the eating of raw fish has been linked to thiamin deficiency.

## Niacin

Niacin (also called nicotinic acid and nicotinamide) has proven the most useful in the treatment of failing memory and confusion that accompanies old age. One of the first documented uses of this vitamin to treat "senile" symptoms was a last-resort experiment by Dr. Abram Hoffer. Concerned by his mother's failing memory and vision at the age of sixty-seven, Hoffer tried giving her large doses of nicotinic acid (a form of niacin)—not because he really thought that the vitamin would be able to improve her memory, but because there was an outside chance that it would produce a beneficial placebo response.

To Hoffer's surprise and delight, his mother began to improve in her mental and physical functioning, and for twenty-one years she continued to take one to four grams of nicotinic acid a day, remaining mentally alert and active, even writing books, until she finally died following a stroke at the age of 88. While one case study hardly represents a scientific sample, we must not overlook the great analytical and intuitive abilities of a researcher of Dr. Hoffer's stature.

Hoffer recommends that any older person who shows depression, anxiety, confusion, and disorientation, should be treated with three grams a day of nicotinic acid; but it is far better, according to Hoffer, to begin nicotinic acid supplementation earlier in life, before there have been any irreversible changes in the brain or the nervous system's biochemistry.

The earlier that an individual begins supplementation with nicotinic acid, the lower will be the dosage required. Hoffer suggests the following preventive dosage schedule (Hoffer and Walker, 1980, p. 145):

| | |
|---|---|
| Age 20–29 | 100 mg. niacin after each meal |
| Age 30–39 | 300 mg. niacin after each meal |
| Age 40–49 | 500 mg. niacin after each meal |
| 50 and over | 1,000 mg. niacin after each meal |

Niacin opens up the tiny blood vessels known as capillaries, bringing a flow of blood to areas long deprived of oxygen and adequate nutrition. While bestowing benefits, this can also induce a "red-hot" sensation just under the skin that can be terrifying!

The amide form of niacin, nicotinamide or niacinamide, will not produce the sometimes unpleasant flushing that is characteristic of this vitamin, but Hoffer believes that older people will derive greater benefits from the nicotinic acid. The optimal dose in any case is that which effectively eliminates symptoms while producing minimal, or no, side effects.

(As a side note, the niacin form is found in plants while niacinamide is found in animal life.)

Hoffer also reports that niacin has another important effect in that it appears to prevent "sludging" of the red blood cells. Red blood cells in some people have a tendency to stick together. Because they are clumped together, the red blood cells cannot travel freely through the tiny capillaries and carry vital oxygen to the tissues.

Such oxygen starvation can obviously have severe effects on mental functioning. Many older people have sludging of the blood and have a characteristic appearance of pale, puffy faces, along with fatigue, tension, and anxiety. When such people are treated with nicotinic acid, they are restored to their normal appearance and their red blood cells no longer clump together. Hoffer reports that anticoagulant drugs that help control sludging are helpful in treating senility and that niacin by itself is a significant antisludging substance. Apparently it works by increasing the negative electrical charge on the red blood cells, so that they repel each other instead of sticking together. (Food sources of this vitamin are given earlier in this chapter.)

## Vitamin B-6

Deficiency symptoms of this vitamin are often seen in the elderly. Irritability, muscular twitchings, even convulsions result when B-6 (pyridoxine) is missing in the diet.

Less traumatic symptoms may occur in early stages of vitamin B-6 deficiency. These include a smooth, red tongue, soreness of the mouth, and a greasy dermatitis around the orbits of the eyes, in the eyebrows, and the corners of the mouth. As the deficiency becomes more pronounced, dizziness, nausea, vomiting, kidney stones, and mental confusion may result. In addition, a reduced state of immunity will occur.

This key vitamin is involved in as many as fifty specific chemical reactions involving the use of amino acids, the starter-compounds of proteins. Of critical importance in brain functions, vitamin B-6 is found in the brain in a concentration of up to twenty-five to fifty times higher than in blood levels! Clearly, the brain and nervous system are highly dependent on this vitamin.

While just 2 milligrams per day is the RDA for vitamin B-6, even this small amount may be missing from the diet of the average person.

Plentiful in whole grains, more than 75 percent of the vitamin is lost in the milling of wheat into white flour. Processing and heating finish the job of destruction. Thus, a diet containing a lot of white bread, pasta, and pre-cooked rice is practically devoid of this vitamin.

To assure an adequate amount of vitamin B-6 be sure to eat wheat germ, sunflower seeds, chickpeas, other nuts, legumes, avocados, bananas, salmon, tuna, and beef (if you are not cholesterol conscious).

## Vitamin B-12

B-12, or cobalamin, is an antistress and antifatigue vitamin that is useful in dealing with general tiredness and nervousness. It was the last vitamin to be discovered and completed the jigsaw puzzle of the B complex.

Known primarily for its role in preventing and treating pernicious anemia, this is the most chemically complicated vitamin. Even if the vitamin is present in the diet, it may be insufficiently absorbed. This malabsorption may be due to a lack of vitamin B-12 binding proteins in the intestines or due to surgical removal of the stomach. It also occurs in people infested with the fish tapeworm, or in people with sprue, tropical anemias, and other conditions of intestinal malabsorption.

Although anemia is rarely seen in an uncomplicated dietary deficiency of this vitamin, a simple deficiency of B-12 will yield symptoms such as back pains, tingling of the extremities, sore tongue, weakness, weight loss, apathy, and other mental abnormalities.

There is *no* vitamin B-12 in plant foods. The richest sources are liver and other organ meats. Next best are meats, fish, eggs, milk, and shellfish. Yogurt provides only a small amount.

The RDA for this vitamin is a low 3 *micro*grams per day, equivalent to that found in one ounce of sardines or herring. For our risk-reduction program, a much higher intake is advised, perhaps 50 to 100 micrograms, as part of a B-complex vitamin tablet.

In summary, the B complex can be very helpful in dealing with the depression, fatigue, and weakness that are so often part of the Alzheimer's disease picture.

## Choline and Lecithin

When students at Northwestern University were given the drug scopolamine, they manifested impairment in memory storage and cognitive functionings that looked like senile behavior, according to Robin Henig in *The Myth of Senility* (Garden City, N.Y.: Anchor Press/Doubleday, 1981, p. 180). Scopolamine interferes with the movement of the nerve-transmitting chemical acetylcholine in the brain. This brain hormone is crucial to the formation of memory. In animal experiments it has been shown that feeding substances rich in choline, which is required for the synthesis of acetylcholine, results in increased amounts of acetylcholine in the hippocampus, the brain's memory center. For this reason, some researchers have recommended an increased dietary intake of choline or lecithin, which contains choline, as a way of promoting proper levels of acetylcholine in the brain.

As reported in a previous chapter, a "long-term, double-blind, placebo-controlled trial of high dose lecithin in senile dementia of the Alzheimer-type" showed a significant improvement in a group of patients who were older than the norm. Drs. Little, Levy, and coworkers were careful to utilize relatively pure lecithin "containing 90 percent phosphatidyl plus lysophosphatidyl choline," at higher dosages than had previously been tried.

Lecithin and choline are of particular interest for someone wishing to reduce the risk of Alzheimer's disease because of their effect on the nervous system. The body manufactures acetylcholine from choline and lecithin in the diet. Acetylcholine is the nerve-transmitting chemical responsible for passing messages from one nerve cell to another in the brain; it regulates the activity of muscles and of the parasympathetic nervous system. It is required for memory, appetite, and sexual behavior and regulates our responsiveness to internal and external stimuli. It controls our ability to "turn off" from the outside environment so we can sleep.

Physical restlessness that prevents sleep, often a problem, may respond to stimulation of acetylcholine production; this can be accomplished by taking choline and lecithin supplements.

A deficiency of acetylcholine can also lead to depression, and hence choline and lecithin can have an antidepressant effect as well as being anxiety-relieving. Because of its calmative effect, lecithin is sometimes used in place of minor tranquilizers.

While there are many lecithin products on the market, two of them are discussed here because physician colleagues mentioned good results with them. Twin Laboratories, Inc. of Ronkonkoma, New York, produces PC-55 which are "antioxidant protected phosphatidyl choline granules." This product contains five times the strength of ordinary lecithin. Lecithin, as it is known in the health trade, contains a mixture of phosphatides. However, most biochemists consider only phosphatidyl choline to be true lecithin. To manufacture this product, TWIN LAB removed the oils from an existing formula resulting in 55% pure phosphatidyl choline lecithin granules. Vitamins C and E have been added to preserve the activity of this lecithin formula.

Another fine product containing acetylcholine precursors is Supercholine[15] manufactured by Cardiovascular Research, Ltd., of Concord, California. Research performed with

15 "Supercholine" and "Free Radical Quenchers" are trademarks of Cardiovascular Research, Ltd. A protocol on brain function and aging may be obtained by writing to the company: CVR, Ltd., 1061-B Shary Circle, Concord CA 94518. (415) 827-2636.

Supercholine at the Neurosciences Research Center, University of Maryland College of Medicine, on patients with Down's syndrome showed a marked improvement in I.Q. scores and other mental parameters, such as memory recall, in patients receiving this valuable dietary supplement. Medical scientists have long noted the striking similarity in the neuropathology of patients with Alzheimer's disease in comparison to Down's syndrome and have repeatedly used Down's patients as a model for senility studies. Using computerized EEG reports (brain wave studies), it was found that patients with deficits in cholinergic function improved following supplementation with this phosphatidyl choline complex.

Supercholine contains pure crystals of all essential phosphatides, including phosphatidylinositol, phoshatidylserine, and phosphatidylethanolamine. A large proportion of "phosphatidylcholine" products commercially available actually contain heated lecithin, which is high in lipid peroxides. Supercholine, since it contains no glycerol or oxidized fatty acids, is devoid of any free radical forming agents.

Pathologists conducting brain tissue biopsies in patients with Alzheimer's disease have found high levels of lipid peroxides (rancid fats) in affected cells. Free radicals induced by lipid peroxides cause nerve cell destruction on a massive scale in susceptible individuals. Fortunately there are ways of minimizing free radical damage to nerve cells through use of dietary antioxidants.

One of the most complete antioxidant formulas available, widely used by physicians in preventive medicine, is "Free Radical Quenchers" (Cardiovascular Research, Ltd., Concord, California). This formula contains high potencies of beta carotene, ascorbyl palmitate (fat-soluble vitamin C),

Vitamin E, lipoic acid, Co-enzyme Q, selenium, and the critical sulfhydryl amino acids: cysteine, methionine, and reduced glutathione.

"Free Radical Quenchers" contains all of the essential precursors of the body's own antioxidant defense network. These antioxidants neutralize the aberrant charge of free radicals in the body and interrupt the chain reactions before cellular death occurs. The brain is particularly susceptible to oxidation reactions and has been identified as the prime target organ.

Disciplined supplementation with the sulfhydryl amino acids and other critical antioxidants, found in "Free Radical Quenchers," serves as an excellent preventive measure in preserving the cellular integrity of the brain and other key organs. Moreover, these antioxidants slow down the aging process of important cell groups in the skin and blood vessels.

As part of our risk-reduction program, adequate amounts of choline should also be derived from foods. It is present in all foods in which phospholipids (i.e. phosphorous connected to fats) are found. These include egg yolk, beef liver, whole grains, legumes, meats, and wheat germ. Soybeans, peas, and beans contain smaller amounts of choline while fruits have little or none of this vitamin. It is not destroyed by heat and remains in dried foods for a long time.

There is no RDA for choline, but a single, one gram capsule of lecithin taken each day, in addition to a multi-vitamin/mineral offers a wise measure of security without the risk of toxicity.

## Vitamin C

Vitamin C plays an important role in combating fatigue, listlessness, confusion, and depression as well as acting as a tranquilizer for the anxious and also helping to relieve insomnia. Thus, vitamin C is an important element of our program, helping to control many of the troublesome symptoms. Vitamin C is so beneficial for these mental symptoms because it plays a key role in the production of neurotransmitters in the brain.

Vitamin C is severely depleted by stress, both mental and physical. In our modern environment, with pollution, psychological stresses, the use of cigarettes, and exposure to other vitamin C-depleting influences, it is no wonder that we require large doses of this truly "miraculous" substance.

People sometimes wonder why large doses of vitamin C should be able to help against such a wide range of problems; perhaps we need to realize that as human beings we need not necessarily be susceptible to infection, slow wound healing, allergies, heart disease, cancer, and mental distress, and that by taking large doses of vitamin C, we are returning to a more normal level of functioning.

Vitamin C has also been shown to reduce serum cholesterol and thus to protect against atherosclerosis. It is a powerful detoxifier, helping to overcome the ill effects of heavy metals, chemicals in air pollution, carcinogenic substances, poisons, and radiation. It also helps combat the undesirable side effects of many medications.

Vitamin C functions as an anticancer agent by combating the formation of cancer-causing chemicals. It not only protects against cancer, but it is also used in high doses to treat certain existing cancers.

It has an important role in stimulating the immune system, helping us to resist disease. It is also important in the formation of collagen, the connective tissue found throughout the body. Collagen is involved in wound healing, which is promoted by vitamin C. Since this vitamin helps maintain the bones, cartilage, and connective tissue, it is an important adjunct to any exercise program, protecting against damage to the spine and joints from jogging and other forms of exercise.

From the perspective of Alzheimer's disease, this vitamin is the "premier free-radical scavenger" according to Robert F. Cathcart III, M.D. Able to "neutralize" toxic compounds, vitamin C serves by protecting cells from oxidation. Known as an antioxidant, this key vitamin therefore may serve to limit or remove "inflammatory, hypersensitivity, and autoimmune conditions," according to Dr. Cathcart (*Medical Hypotheses*, 18: 1985).

A current theory relates the possible breakdown of the immune system to the onset of Alzheimer's disease. If Dr. Cathcart is correct, vitamin C, in sufficient dosage, will act to prevent antigens from attaching to antibodies. This essentially stops the inflammation seen in allergic reactions, but may also explain why patients generally experience speedier recovery from viral illnesses when they utilize this vitamin.

For the elderly and infirm, especially those in nursing homes (and thus inactive), vitamin C can be a critical component both in preventing and limiting the course of infections. Simply its capacity to raise resistance to infections is reason enough to assure adequate intake of vitamin C.

For maintenance, I recommend 1-2 grams per day. In disease states, use enough vitamin C to achieve "bowel tolerance," or until you experience gas or diarrhea, and then reduce this amount by 10 percent to achieve your effective dose.

## Vitamin E

One of the most notable functions of vitamin E, in terms of brain function, is its ability to facilitate the transport of oxygen to the blood. Vitamin E is a crucial part of our program, helping to fight fatigue and oxygen starvation in the cells to produce a nontoxic, natural state of alertness. Vitamin E is intimately related to aerobic exercise. The more intense the exercise, the higher is the requirement for this vitamin.

Vitamin E is a very effective antioxidant and free radical deactivator, protecting the structural integrity of the cell membranes and helping neutralize the damaging effect of smog and other environmental pollutants, including the carbon monoxide in cigarette smoke. It is the only known antioxidant that protects cellular structures by preventing lipid peroxidation—the breakdown of fatty substances.

Vitamin E also appears to prevent the accumulation of cholesterol in the arteries and protects against the formation of abnormal blood clots, which can result in heart attack or stroke.

It is reported to have a calming effect on nervous or exhausted individuals and has helped to relieve the mental symptoms of menopause. One of its earliest discovered functions was the prevention of sterility in rats, and, although its reputation as a "sex vitamin" was exaggerated, it does help protect the sex hormones as well as other substances in the body against oxidation.

Vitamin E is most effective when it is taken with other antioxidants, such as the mineral selenium, vitamin C, and the amino acid cystine. It should be taken with meals that contain some fats or oils since these are necessary to induce bile flow, which is necessary in order for the vitamin E to be properly assimilated.

Vitamin E deficiency produces a breakage of red blood cell membranes, which supports our strong recommendations for adequate intake of this cell-saving nutrient. In point of fact, current aging theory addresses the cell membrane as a critical element in the aging process. By preventing cell membrane damage, vitamin E slows the road to debility and demise. (Interestingly, muscular dystrophy in animals can be produced by feeding a diet deficient in vitamin E!)

Since this vitamin is carried in the blood through its attachment to lipoproteins, you must eat a diet with sufficient fats and proteins to receive its benefits.

The major sources of vitamin E in the diet are vegetable and, now, fish oils. The rest of our dietary supply comes from whole grains, liver, beans, fruits, and vegetables. Almonds and peanuts are especially good sources of this all-saving, antiaging nutrient and should be freely served to those following our risk-reduction program. A dosage range of between 150-400 I.U. is generally recommended as safe.

## The Minerals

### Calcium/Magnesium

One of the troublesome symptoms of elderly people is muscle cramping and twitching. These symptoms are relieved by the minerals calcium and magnesium, which act as natural tranquilizers and muscle relaxants.

Calcium is the most plentiful mineral element in the body. Most of it goes to make up our bones and teeth, while a very small proportion of calcium in the soft tissues and blood has a crucial effect on nerve function. Extreme calcium deficiency can produce twitching of the muscles, cramps, irritation, confusion, even convulsions; while lesser degrees of deficiency can result in depression, irritability, impaired memory, and calf cramps.

Magnesium acts as a natural tranquilizer for the nervous system and has been used to treat anxiety, depression, insomnia, and hyperactivity in children. It is also essential for normal heart function. It regulates the critical balance of various substances in the body, such as sodium and chloride, calcium, and phosphorus.

Calcium and magnesium should be taken in the ratio of 1:1. If there is too much or too little magnesium in relation to calcium, the body may not absorb enough calcium.

Current advertising coming from certain drug companies promotes calcium consumption, *without* the support of magnesium! The long-term effects on the millions of women now gobbling antacids as a calcium supplement may very well be the deposit of calcium along arterial walls, not in the bones. Worse, many of these heavily advertised antacids contain relatively large quantities of *aluminum*!

Therefore, do not take your calcium from antacids and make certain that the supplement you buy has an *equal* amount of magnesium. If this is not possible (many formulas contain these minerals in a ratio of 2:1), simply take an *additional* quantity of magnesium to equal your intake of the supplementary calcium.

Remember also that adequate, NOT excess, *protein* is vital to calcium absorption. Too much protein actually causes calcium loss! The RDA for an average adult calls for just two to three ounces of lean protein per day. Any more than this will be wasted and pull valuable calcium out of circulation.

Meat contains phosphorous that, in excess, blocks calcium utilization, which makes it a *poor* protein choice. Soft cola drinks also contain phosphorous (in the form of "phosphoric acid") and must be avoided for proper calcium metabolism. Remember too, that dairy products contain calcium but very little magnesium to help absorb the calcium.

Losses of magnesium occur whenever you take a diuretic (to promote water loss), drink excess coffee, tea, or alcohol.

There are good sources of magnesium, the silvery-white trace metal so essential for the high-energy transfers going on in our cells. Wheat bran, wheat germ, coffee, cocoa, brewer's yeast, black walnuts, roasted peanuts, whole wheat products, raw beet greens, even chocolate contain magnesium in descending order. Other good food sources are green, leafy vegetables.

Animal products such as milk and meat are fairly *poor* sources of magnesium. Processing destroys much of this mineral so next to nothing remains in rice and white pasta. Boiling vegetables causes great losses, so save the water and use it in soups, gravies, etc. Sugar, alcohol, fats, and oils contain almost no magnesium.

The RDA for this mineral is about 350 milligrams per day. You can get this much from nuts, seeds, cocoa, coffee, fruits, and legumes. (Three ounces of walnuts or peanuts yields about two thirds of the RDA). If you take a calcium supplement more magnesium will be required.

Earlier in this book we mentioned how the disease ALS, found in many people in the regions of Guam, New Guinea, and Japan, is related to locales where the water and soil is deficient in calcium and magnesium. Since this neurological disease shares many similarities with Alzheimer's disease it is worth quoting an expert who studied sufferers of ALS directly.

"Analysis of drinking water from three wells and of soil from the gardens and villages of ALS patients reveals extremely low calcium and magnesium, with relatively high silicon, iron, titanium, chromium and aluminum....Dr. Yase has suggested that calcium and magnesium deficiency and an excess of aluminum and manganese in the Guam and Kii foci is responsible for the high incidence of ALS ... and the early appearance of neurofibrillary tangles in the populations." (D. Gajdusek, M.D., Laboratory of Central Nervous System Studies, National Institutes of Health, Bethesda, Maryland; In: Chen and Yase, 1984; 145-55.) Essentially, when we do not take in adequate quantities of calcium and magnesium, our bodies accept other minerals in their place. When excess aluminum is present, this toxic metal is absorbed and slowly deposited in nerve cells. The end result of a lifetime of such an imbalance can be Alzheimer's disease.

## Zinc

Of the mineral nutrients that can help to prevent senile changes in the nervous system, the most important are zinc and magnesium. Zinc is essential to the synthesis of RNA, DNA, and protein and to the maintenance of vitamin A levels in the blood. Zinc deficiency can cause a confusional state in the elderly and can produce a decrease in the senses of smell and taste. When older people are not eating properly, zinc deficiency may be at fault since food is less appetizing when the senses of smell and taste are reduced.

The old wives' tale about masturbation bringing about insanity has a possible link with current knowledge in nutritional science. Dr. Carl Pfeiffer, of the Brain Bio Center in Princeton, New Jersey, explains that about 2 or more milligrams of zinc are lost during extended intercourse. (See his "Mental and Elemental Nutrients." New Canaan, Conn.: Keats Publishing Co., 1975.)

Some men who are very active sexually, or masturbate to excess, also consume diets inadequate in this critical trace metal, which is utilized in the creation of sperm, seminal fluid, and many hormones. Such loss in an already zinc-depleted male could possibly produce psychological symptoms, as Dr. Pfeiffer observes:

> "Perhaps with zinc-deficient males, some degree of nervousness and even psychosis might result from excessive masturbation, but since the female loses little by way of secretions with masturbation, the old nineteenth-century diagnosis of masturbatory

> insanity could scarcely be applied accurately to women." (Pfeiffer 1975, p. 471)

Even if you don't fear insanity, it is a good idea to take extra zinc because most of our soils are depleted of this trace metal. The best food sources are oysters, shellfish, fish, whole grains (especially oatmeal), eggs, legumes, and nuts. Pumpkin seeds are particularly zinc-rich and are recommended regularly by European physicians who know that prostatitis can be controlled or reversed with zinc. Be sure that your vitamin/mineral pill plus food sources adds up to at least 30 milligrams, or else supplement with a separate zinc tablet.

## Selenium

Selenium, another mineral element in our program, can be highly poisonous in too-high doses. Because the toxic dose is very close to the dose for dietary supplementation, nutritionists have been very cautious in recommending selenium as a supplement. However, we now know that it is an extremely important trace mineral, acting as an antioxidant as does vitamin E, and a free radical deactivator. It slows down aging, prevents heart and blood vessel disease, and may help to prevent cancer (Shamberger, 1969).

Adequate selenium is required in order for vitamin E to perform many of its functions. It enhances the efficiency of vitamin E, while at the same time vitamin E increases the body's tolerance to the potentially toxic selenium. Besides their antioxidant and anti-free radical activity, vitamin E and selenium together also improve the functioning of the immune system, boosting resistance to disease. Working with other antioxidants, selenium can be a crucial part of an Alzheimer's risk-reduction program.

Food sources include garlic, asparagus, seafood, meat, and grains grown on selenium-containing soils. Very little is found in fruits and vegetables.

The proposed RDA for this powerful antioxidant will be between 50 to 200 *micro*grams per day, about equal to that consumed in typical American diets. Selenium can be toxic above 600 micrograms per day (loss of hair and nails is an early symptom), so supplementation above 50 mcg. per day is *not* advisable.

## The Amino Acids

### Cystine (an anti-toxicant)

Cystine is one of the sulfur-containing amino acids. This amino acid serves an important protective function and should be part of our risk-reduction program. It contains the sulfhydryl group (an atom of sulfur and an atom of hydrogen), which is a component of the important metabolite Coenzyme A, which participates in a great many vital reactions in the body.

Cystine helps to destroy harmful chemicals in the body such as acetaldehyde and free radicals produced by smoking, drinking, and accelerated metabolic processes. Thus, it works with the vitamin and mineral antioxidants and free radical scavengers to protect against damage from free radical action. It also helps to prevent brain and liver damage from alcohol and protects against radiation, heavy metals, and other harmful substances in the body.

It appears also that cystine is necessary for the proper utilization of vitamin B-6. A number of chronic degenerative diseases, both mental and physical, seem to be caused by a disorder in the utilization of B-6; hence the real, underlying cause of these diseases may be a cystine deficiency.

Cystine is considered a "nonessential" amino acid because it can be formed within the body from the essential amino acid methionine. It is found in all good protein foods such as egg white, milk, fish, meat, legumes, rice, and other common food items.

Supplements are not necessary if the diet contains an adequate quantity of high-quality protein, about two to three ounces per day.

## Glutamine

*Glutamic* acid, one of the "nonessential" amino acids, has a unique function in brain metabolism. It is the only substance other than glucose that can serve as a fuel for the brain, and so it has been shown to give a lift from fatigue and improve intelligence, among other benefits. Glutamic acid also protects the body by serving as a buffer against excess ammonia, in what is known as the "citric acid cycle."

Although glutamic acid provides energy for the brain, it isn't possible for the brain to derive glutamic acid directly from food, owing to the protective blood-brain barrier that allows only a very few chemicals to enter the brain directly from the blood.

However, it is possible to increase the glutamic acid in the brain by providing the proper building blocks in the diet. Besides its function as a source of energy for the brain, glutamine has also been shown to protect against the poisonous effects of alcohol and to stop a craving for alcohol. Studies have shown that glutamine helps to fight fatigue, depression, and impotence, and it has been used successfully against schizophrenia, senility, and mental retardation in limited trials.

Richard Kunin, M.D., a psychiatrist well versed in nutritional medicine, recently communicated his concerns regarding this amino acid. He writes "Amino acids are not without dangers when used in therapeutics. Glutamic acid and glutamine add to the ammonia burden, which can aggravate neurotoxicity in some susceptible people." (Personal communication, 1986.)

Again, eating good quality protein foods is the safest course of action for our risk-reduction program.

## Phenylalanine

The amino acid *phenylalanine* creates a natural sense of well being, owing to its role in producing the nerve transmitting chemicals adrenaline and noradrenaline, as well as other important hormones. This nutrient appears to help overcome depression, increase mental alertness, improve memory, control allergies, and aid weight loss by suppressing appetite.

The body's requirement for phenylalanine is higher than for the other amino acids. It is the raw material that produces several compounds known as catecholamines-neurotransmitters, which include adrenaline and noradrenaline. The adrenal medulla and the nerve cells can manufacture these catecholamines only when there is enough phenylalanine (or its derivative, tyrosine) in the blood. Adrenaline and noradrenaline are responsible for a positive, elevated mood of alertness.

Medical researchers have often tried to produce this state of alertness through the use of drugs such as amphetamines. However, such an artificial manipulation ultimately leads to an aggravation of the original depression. It is a more natural solution to provide adequate levels of dietary phenylalanine, thereby assuring that normal levels of noradrenaline will be maintained in the brain and nerves, providing a boost in energy and alertness that is not followed by a "crash."

Again, we are cautioned against taking phenylalanine as a supplement by Dr. Kunin. This amino acid "is likely to cause neurotoxicity in people with subclinical or a recessive form of phenylketonuria and they should not take supplements."

## Tyrosine

*Tyrosine* is another amino acid that helps to overcome depression, increase mental alertness, and improve memory. Like phenylalanine, tyrosine is involved in the manufacture of the neuro-transmitters adrenaline and noradrenaline, which are responsible for an elevated, positive mood.

If there is sufficient phenylalanine in the body, the liver can manufacture adequate tyrosine from the phenylalanine.

In one study (Gelenberg, A., 1980. "Tyrosine for the Treatment of Depression." *Amer. J. Psy.*, 147-62), tyrosine supplementation was shown to control anxiety and long-standing depression; patients who had previously been treated for these problems with amphetamines were able to discontinue or reduce their dosage of the drugs.

Allergy sufferers and those on weight-loss programs have also had positive responses to tyrosine, which is a much preferred way to control appetite as opposed to the use of amphetamines or other "diet pills."

However, if used as a supplement, it should be done so under proper medical supervision.

## Tryptophan (a natural sedative)

Unlike the "psychic energizers" glutamine, phenylalanine, and tyrosine, the amino acid tryptophan has a calming effect on the nervous system. Tryptophan is well known for its ability to alleviate insomnia. It reduces anxiety, depression, and pain as well as improves sleep. (All critical in the aged.)

Tryptophan works as a building block for the neurotransmitter serotonin. In an experiment, cats deprived of brain serotonin became insomniacs! Unlike drugs used to treat insomnia and anxiety, tryptophan does not suppress central nervous system functioning but rather restores normal function by being available for the body to use in making serotonin as needed.

Tryptophan has other important functions as well. Recently it has been discovered that heart attacks are often triggered by irregular heartbeats or arterial spasms due to a lack of serotonin. For this reason adequate intake of tryptophan can conceivably reduce the risk of this type of heart attack, which accounts for more than 15 percent of heart disease deaths, by making the heart less susceptible to stress-induced changes.

Some tryptophan is used to make the B vitamin niacin in people who are deficient in this vitamin. Therefore, you should maintain an adequate intake of niacin if you want to get the full benefit of the tryptophan; this is accomplished by taking the B complex and multivitamin supplements recommended.

Eating complex carbohydrate-dense foods will lead to an elevation of tryptophan in the blood. So a large plate of pasta, rice, or potatoes is a natural way to induce a state of calm. Milk, too, is rich in this amino acid. The custom of having a glass of *warm* milk before bedtime is wise; the heat frees the tryptophan and enables it to be rapidly absorbed. By eventually elevating blood levels of serotonin, the natural tranquilizer, a peaceful sleep is induced.

## How to Buy a Multivitamin/Mineral Formula

This is the backbone of your nutrient therapy and should be selected with great care. Do not buy a discount or supermarket multivitamin. Stick to a reputable manufacturer. The cheap brands often fail to deliver adequate quantities of nutrients and rely on poor quality ingredients. In addition, they often contain fillers, binders, colorings, and other questionable additives.

### Here Is How to Select Your Brand:

1. How much Vitamin E does it contain? This is the most expensive ingredient in a "multi" and often in short supply. A good formula will contain at least 150 I.U. of *mixed* tocopherols. Read the label carefully. If the brand contains "*alpha*-tocopherol" you are only getting a *portion* of the vitamin E required. Only "mixed tocopherols" assure you of the whole vitamin E complex.
2. *Biotin*: Make sure it contains at least 100 mcg. (micrograms). This is another highly expensive

nutrient (often omitted from discount brands) and a good indicator of the general quality of your overall formula. It is essential in forming nucleic acids, glycogen, and required in the synthesis of several amino acids.

3. *Chromium*: It should contain between 100-200 mcg. of this mineral, which is of critical importance in proper functioning of glucose and carbohydrate metabolism. This trace mineral has a key role, as part of the "glucose-tolerance-factor," or GTF, in preventing and controlling adult-onset diabetes.
4. *Selenium*: Make sure your multi contains 20 to 50 mcg. of this antioxidant. The safe limit is about 100-200 mcg. daily, including food sources.
5. Of course the multi you select will also contain other nutrients. I have listed those that are the keys to evaluating a superior formula.

Be sure to take this "backbone" vitamin/mineral formula every day. Then build upon it with the full range of supplements recommended. Of course, supplements are just that. They are meant to supplement foods, not replace them,

By eating the foods specified for each nutrient discussed in this chapter you will be doing a great deal toward reducing your risk of Alzheimer's disease.

**An Ideal "Multi" Formula**[16]
MaxiLIFE® $CoQ_{10}$ FORMULA
Multiple Vitamin Mineral
Manufactured by TWIN LABORATORIES, INC.
RONKONKOMA, NEW YORK 11779 U.S.A.

| NUTRIENT | DOSAGE | % U.S. RDA |
|---|---|---|
| Four capsules supply: | | |
| $CoQ_{10}$ (coenzyme $Q_{10}$) | 30 mg. | * |
| Dry Vitamin A Acetate (water dispersed) | 5,000 I.U. | 100 |
| Dry Vitamin D-3 (water dispersed) | 200 I.U. | 50 |
| Dry Beta-Carotene (water dispersed) | 25,000 I.U. | 500 |
| Dry Vitamin E (d-alpha tocopheryl succinate) | 400 I.U | 1333 |
| Vitamin C | 1,000 mg. | 1666 |
| Ascorbyl Palmitate (fat soluble vitamin C—42 mg. as vitamin C) | 100 mg. | 70 |
| Citrus Bioflavonoid Complex | 100 mg. | * |
| Vitamin B-l | 25 mg. | 1666 |
| Vitamin B-2 | 25 mg. | 1470 |
| Vitamin B-6 | 75 mg. | 3750 |
| Vitamin B-3 (niacinamide) | 125 mg. | 625 |
| Pantothenic Acid | 100 mg. | 1000 |
| Vitamin B-12 | 100 mcg. | 1666 |
| Folic Acid | 800 mcg. | 200 |
| Biotin | 300 mcg. | 100 |
| PABA | 10 mg. | * |
| Choline Bitartrate | 225 mg. | * |
| Inositol | 100 mg. | * |
| Calcium (from calcium carbonate & citrate) | 50 mg. | 5 |
| Magnesium (from magnesium aspartate & oxide) | 100 mg. | 25 |
| Potassium (from potassium chloride) | 10 mg. | * |
| Zinc (from chelated zinc citrate) | 30 mg. | 200 |

16 We have selected this formula as the most complete. Also it does not contain iron, which is wise, owing to its ability to destroy protective nutrients.

| | | |
|---|---|---|
| Manganese (from chelated manganese gluconate) | 5 mg. | * |
| Copper[17] (from coated chelated copper gluconate) | 2 mg. | 100 |
| Iodine (from potassium iodide) | 150 mcg. | 100 |
| Selenium (from yeast free selenomethionine & selenate) | 200 mcg. | * |
| Chromium (from yeast free trivalent chromium) | 200 mcg. | * |
| Molybdenum (from natural molybdic acid) | 250 mcg. | * |
| L-Cysteine | 250 mg. | * |
| L-Methionine | 100 mg. | * |
| L-Glutathione | 50 mg. | * |

* No U.S. RDA has been established.

17 Specially coated to prevent interaction with incompatible nutrients.

## Conclusions

# THE ALUMINUM CONNECTION

We have seen that many theories exist to explain Alzheimer's disease, and unifying these diverse theories are *malnutrition* on the one hand with an excessive intake of aluminum on the other.

We can limit our intake of this toxic metal by adjusting our food consumption, our use of drugs, and the cookware we use. By eating foods that contain sulfhydryl groups, such as egg yolks, garlic, onion, beans, and others, we can rid ourselves of some of the aluminum and other toxic metals we may take in. And, we can establish a risk-reduction diet by learning from the people of Vilcabamba, Ecuador, who eat foods of the kind suggested in this book, especially those rich in calcium and magnesium. We have also seen how their consistent *endurance* type of activities disposes them toward healthful longevity.

Many of us now practice *intense* exercise. Yet, this is not as beneficial as the *duration* of our activities. The long-lived people of Ecuador, and of other regions studied in some detail, all remain physically active throughout their lives. Endurance types of activities, such as walking, bicycling, jogging, aerobics, swimming, skiing, and rowing more closely approximate the type of physical activities engaged in by our long-lived models, who scarcely exert themselves, preferring instead consistent activity of long endurance.

Such types of physical activity act toward *chelating* toxic *metals*, such as aluminum, removing them from our systems. This is owing to the *lactic acid* formed during exercise. The lactate in our blood is a good chelating agent, and the amount produced is "more dependent on the *duration* of the muscular exertion, than on its *intensity* ... endurance type activities," both elevating and *maintaining*, lactic acid levels in our blood. (J. Bjorksten, 1980, and other references he cites).

It is for this reason that the type of diet explained in this book, in conjunction with endurance activities and an aluminum-elimination program, all work to reduce the risk of developing Alzheimer's disease.

When Alzheimer's disease strikes a victim, it has been found that the families themselves meet almost 50 percent of the expenses from their own funds. Thus, a family member with Alzheimer's disease can represent a terrible drain on his family's financial, as well as emotional, resources. Diagnostic evaluation of a patient, alone, may cost between $300 and $2,000.

Alzheimer's disease is also a drain on federal reserves, with an estimated federal expenditure for long-term care in 1985 of $24 billion. By 1990, it is estimated that the figure will be $43 billion, and Alzheimer's disease will probably account for around 50 percent of these funds.

For those of us who wish to prevent this disease, the risk-reduction program offers a sound, scientific approach, readily enacted. For those suffering from this illness, the program outlined can do no harm. Instead it offers a positive, inexpensive plan of action where little now exists.

# Afterword

On the very day I was preparing to send to my publisher the final, copyedited version of the manuscript for this book, I learned of a discovery that seemed to relate to my risk-reduction program.

During a telephone discussion with a scientist at the National Institutes of Health, I was privileged to learn of the discovery of the gene for the development of amyloid, an abnormal protein found in the cells of Alzheimer's disease patients. What puzzled me was the discovery that this gene is found in everybody! Why its coding for developing this abnormal protein took effect in some, but not all, people was an interesting question.

After some reflection I realized that a neurotoxic agent, such as aluminum, could possibly "trigger" this gene, in addition to making specific brain cells vulnerable to the development of amyloid directly. A lifetime of calcium and magnesium deficiencies could permit brain cells to incorporate the aluminum-protein complexes seen in the disease.

This discovery of the gene for producing amyloid may be seized upon as "the answer" to the Alzheimer's disease riddle, especially by those who choose not to *arrive* at a rational conclusion more carefully. Whether this disease is brought about by a poor genetic inheritance or triggered by environmental events will be debated with some heat.

The "nature vs. nurture" debate has polarized the biological sciences for decades. A controversy such as this has always divided scientists into two opposing groups: one that believes "it's all in the genes," the other group that the *environment* influences the manifestation of a disease.

I firmly believe that both nature *and* nurture are involved in system expressions, especially in many diseases. In the case of Alzheimer's disease, the discovery of a gene for producing amyloid is less revolutionary than it might at first appear. This gene appears in humans without regard to whether or not Alzheimer's disease has appeared. It is universal.

This clearly indicates that *other factors* are required to have the abnormal protein peculiar to Alzheimer's disease develop. This discovery also demonstrates that we should be able to influence those environmental factors likely to be responsible for the initiation and development of the disease—notably the complex mineral imbalance that seems to be implicated.

While the entire story of this new discovery remains to be told, I believe my risk-reduction program to be the best available answer we now have for the prevention of this disease.

Port Washington
January 1987

## Continuing Research

Since the publication of the first edition, a growing body of evidence further supports the role of aluminum in Alzheimer's disease and the nutritional interventions which are useful in combatting the disease.

Aluminum has been known as a neurotoxic substance for nearly a century and the scientific literature on its toxic effects has now grown to a critical mass. We are *not* saying that aluminum *causes* Alzheimer's. It is, however, the only element noted to accumulate in the neurofibrillary tangles which are characteristic of the disease. While this evidence does not prove that aluminum caused the plaques (the aluminum-containing masses found in the brain of Alzheimer's patients), it does add weight to the concept that aluminum plays an early role in plaque formation. The famous British study of aluminum in drinking water by Martyn, et al., published in *The Lancet*, is further evidence that "chronic low exposure can lead to deposition inside neurons in the brain" (as reported in *Chemistry and Industry*, June 6, 1988, p. 346).

The Martyn study has been criticized for a number of "methodological problems," but we agree with the conclusion that "the relative risk of having Alzheimer's was related to the concentration of aluminum in the water."

We also know that "some, if not all, cases of Alzheimer's disease are linked to a mutation in the proximal portion of the long arm of chromosome 21 ..." As D. R. McLachlan and co-workers at the University of Toronto Faculty of Medicine further postulate, "one consequence of the mutation is loss of the natural barriers and intracellular ligands for aluminum. As a result, aluminum gains access to several brain sites including the nuclear compartment in certain neurons of the central nervous system." (Personal communication, in press.)

In a recent communication, Dr. W. J. Lukiw of the University of Toronto (Canada), Centre for Research in Neurodegenerative Diseases, informs us that an *in vitro* simulation of Alzheimer's disease confirms that aluminum negatively influences genetic function (Lukiw, 1987). He further states "our paper entitled 'Linker Histone—DNA Completes ...', to be published in Federation of European Bichemical Societies (FEBS) circa September or October 1989, also substantiates the claim that aluminum basically 'gums up' chromatin at very basic levels of genomic organization." As he and Drs. Kruck and McLachlan stated in their 1987 paper, all the evidence would "suggest an aluminum induced impairment in the readout of the genetic information."

It will be only a short time before the medical establishment accepts the implications of this evidence. At that time, many people will choose to eliminate aluminum from their diets just as they now eschew cholesterol-laden foods. The readers of this book need not wait twenty or more years, however, to begin making changes which can vastly improve brain health.

Those who remain skeptical regarding the evidence which supports the protocol presented in Chapters 4-7 should refer to the article published in *The Lancet*, January 14, 1989, page 59-62, by C. N. Martyn and colleagues. This is the strongest of the *five* epidemiological studies which have been published on the role of aluminum in drinking water in Alzheimer's disease.

There is also increasing evidence that aluminum in *antacids* may pose an even greater risk, owing to the degree of bioavailability of aluminum in these products. Dr. Laura Fleming and associates discuss this concern in *The Lancet*, February 25, 1989, page 433, concluding in part ". . . there should be an even stronger correlation between Alzheimer's disease and the long-term use of antacids containing aluminum."

With regard to the efficacy of choline, interested skeptics should review the landmark article by A. Little, et al, in the *Journal of Neurology, Neurosurgery, and Psychiatry*, 1985: volume 48, pages 736-742. This study, "A Double Blind, Placebo Controlled Trial of High Dose Lecithin In Alzheimer's Disease," indicated that with high quality choline, in *dosages higher* than those tried previously, a significant number of patients enjoyed a restoration of memory and other cognitive functions.

## How Metals Promote Free-Radical Formation Damaging Brain Cells

We know that metals damage brain cells by promoting the formation of free-radical compounds from hydrogen peroxide. In certain regions of the brain, especially in the basal ganglia, a type of brain cell, excessive amounts of hydrogen peroxide are formed. When this compound contacts certain reduced transitional metals (such as iron and copper) free-radicals are formed which damage brain cell membranes (Dr. M. B. H.

Youdim, Department of Pharmacology, Faculty of Medicine, Technion Israel Institute of Technology, 1988).

"Metals have always been implicated in the pathogenesis of neurologic and psychiatric disorders. Parkinson's disease and Alzheimer's disease have not escaped such scrutiny because metals promote the formation of excess and highly reactive free radicals, which in turn can induce membrane fluidity and degeneration by a process of lipid peroxidation. Such a phenomenon has on several occasions been implicated as intimately involved in these two neurodegenerative disorders." (Youdim, 1988.)

While iron can promote such membrane lipid peroxidation, aluminum does not have such an effect. Nevertheless, "aluminum has extensive synergistic action (1500%) on the lipid peroxidation induced by iron" (Youdim, 1988).

While the above synergism has been demonstrated in vitro only, we must not overlook the interactions between iron and aluminum in Alzheimer's disease.

While awaiting the outcome of such studies, we can take affirmative steps to protect our brain cells thereby reducing our risk of Alzheimer's disease. For example, it is well established that Vitamin C occurs in high concentrations in the basal ganglia. This vitamin blocks the formation of harmful free-radical compounds and, acting as an antioxidant, protects the membranes of our brain cells. Interestingly, in the brains of Parkinson's disease sufferers significant decreases of Vitamin C and glutathione have been noted. This observation "led Perry, et al. to suggest that Parkinson's disease may be a disorder associated with glutathione deficiency of substantia nigra. MPTP, the dopaminergic Parkinson-inducing neurotoxin, causes depletion of glutathione in the substantia nigra, which is prevented by pretreatment with the antioxidant ascorbic acid. The morphologic and biochemical changes induced by MPTP and buthionine sulfoxine, and intracellular inhibitor of glutathione, are remarkably similar." (Youdim, 1988).

These and other studies clearly indicate the role of antioxidants such as Vitamin C in retarding or even preventing the progression of Parkinson's disease and Alzheimer's disease. In addition to using Vitamin C and other antioxidants, aluminum-chelating substances such as desferrioxamine, which is ion-specific to aluminum and which crosses the blood-brain barrier, may also be utilized in an overall Alzheimer's risk reduction program.

## Evolution and the Natural Selection of Trace Elements

It is necessary to understand how the selection of one trace element over another by man and other animals has spelled the difference between evolutionary success or failure. This will serve to further emphasize how *our* selection of trace elements, through foods and supplements, may also determine the status of our brain functions, especially memory and the speed of processing.

Evolutionary choices were made as life evolved from the sea. Selection for survival would depend upon these choices, but the evolving organisms could not know this in advance, if they could "know" at all! Some organisms made the right evolutionary choices, by using, in this case, the elements available to succeed and thus to continue evolving. Some succeeded in part only, utilizing some of the "right" and some of the "wrong" elements. These mediocre creatures ended in evolutionary stasis. Some failed, becoming extinct. "Success depended upon the right choices made at the right time." (H. A. Schroeder)

As vertebrates left the sea for dry land, they carried their chemical systems intact. Their macro and micro trace element balance was evolutionarily fixed. In the primeval seas, they had found their perfect balance of trace elements; some would stay there, complacent in the environment in which they had evolved.

Other creatures, destined for great thrusts on evolution's canvas, were *not* complacent. By choice or by force, they invaded the land.

Going back to the amniotic fluid of all living creatures—the sea—let us examine a choice or two which led to a blind-end of the road or *cul de sac* for some organisms.

Copper was selected by most mollusks for their oxidation-reduction systems and for carrying oxygen in their blood, but this trace metal has severe disadvantages for this task. It has only half the oxygen-carrying capacity of iron. "Copper protein complexes are found in the blood of mollusks, arthropods and trilobites, and was widely used by many animals in the Paleozoic era." Crustaceans also chose copper.

Those mollusks which selected iron to carry their blood oxygen are capable of living out of water. Snails, for example, slithered from the seas and made their way to dry land.

Fortunately for us, "worms chose *iron* to carry their blood oxygen; being twice as efficient, it allowed the evolution of the vertebrates ending in that prime vertebrate of all, Man."

This choice of iron as a blood-oxygen carrier element initiated a series of other revolutionary processes, processes which have brought us to the present state in our evolutionary pathway and which must be seen from the perspective of both positive and negative trace metals.

Zinc, we know, is intimately involved in numerous brain activities, including memory. As a group IIB trace metal, zinc occurs with cadmium and mercury. But whereas zinc is a beneficial trace metal, cadmium is harmful and can interfere with various enzyme systems which require zinc. With sufficient zinc, cadmium will be blocked and it will not displace zinc in the body. By eating foods which contain more than normal quantities of cadmium and less than normal quantities of zinc, cadmium slowly accumulates in the tissues, leading to numerous disorders.

Likewise with aluminum, when we do not receive adequate quantities of calcium and magnesium and we take in aluminum, this toxic trace metal tends to accumulate in the tissues, especially in brain tissue.

Enough is known about Alzheimer's disease to predict with a high degree of certainty that once aluminum is deposited in brain cells, especially those found in the hippocampal region, memory and other functions diminish. To preserve our memory, we must look at those elements which help and those which harm.

## Magnetism May Affect Brain Activity

From the viewpoint of theoretical gerontology another hypothesis may be important. Tadanobu Tsunoda, in his brilliant book "The Japanese Brain" (just translated into English), states that "the addition of a magnetic influence....can affect test results [of brain function]. Therefore, a change taking place on a global scale or even on a cosmic scale at present may be causing a variation in the magnetic field of the earth, affecting brain activity."

Knowing that a magnetic field can affect brain activity leads one to wonder what effects high voltage electrical fields, caused by common electric utility transmission lines, are causing on the human brain. More specifically, might such magnetic fields affect the migration of various trace metals within the human body? Can, for example, proximity to such magnetic fields for extended periods of time cause iron, aluminum, and magnesium to alter their normal course through cells, thus augmenting the deposition of neurotoxic aluminum in neurons?

## Aluminum and Dietary Factors in Alzheimer's Disease

The Fund for Ethnic Medicine[18] has, as a public service, undertaken a dietary epidemiological study of aluminum and protective nutrients in their relation to Alzheimer's disease.

## Study Summary

In our study of the relationship between aluminum, other metallic elements, protective nutrients and Alzheimer's disease, two hundred twenty-seven (227) people *without* any symptoms of the disease were interviewed. All were over 60 years of age. A self-programmed retrospective dietary ques-

18 The Fund for Ethnic Medicine is a California not-for-profit corporation unencumbered by governmental, political, or corporate ties. Through private support including the foresight and generosity of Eric and Sal Estorick of London, England, novel biomedical research is conducted. Inquiries may be directed to FEM, Box 2056, San Rafael, California 94912-2056.

tionnaire was supplied and later reviewed by an epidemiologist with training in human nutrition.

Several interesting patterns appear to be operant in this population.

1. These "brain-healthy" people self-scored a relative "high" or "medium" intake of all 4 nutrients known to protect brain function (choline, vitamin B12, niacin, and folic acid). Iron, which may play a paradoxical role in Alzheimer's disease, was consumed in "high" or "medium" quantities only by 14% of the study population. (See Table 1.)
2. Of the people who consumed alcohol between "one or more" and "three or more" times per week (50% of the respondents), the greatest number consumed wine three or more times per week. Interestingly, beer was consumed by a significantly minute percentage of these seniors without Alzheimer's disease. Beer in aluminum cans may be a factor in the Alzheimer's disease riddle. (See Table 2.)
3. Forty-nine percent (49%) of these brain-healthy people had taken a multi-vitamin preparation for an average of 17 years; 42% took a vitamin C supplement for an average of 15 years and 21% took a B-complex supplement for an average of 16 years.
4. Surprisingly, minerals and other nutrients thought to influence brain-function were *not* taken as supplements by any significant number of the study population. (See Table 3.)

5. A significant number of people reportedly took antacids and buffered aspirin for many years. Known to contain significant quantities of aluminum, it appears that these preparations may be self-limiting in their contribution to the overall aluminum load; or, the intake of vitamin supplements and other protective factors may block the uptake of aluminum into brain cells. (Table 4.)
6. Eighty-five percent (85%) of the respondents used some caffeine-containing beverage on a regular basis. Apparently, caffeine does *not* appear to be implicated in Alzheimer's disease. (Table 5.)
7. It appears that food containing aluminum may offer sufficient protection against aluminum absorption, either as a result of nutrients they contain (such as calcium) or by slowing the absorption of aluminum in another manner. (Table 6.)
8. Respondents ascribed certain factors for their good health; namely, diet, exercise and genetics. As respondents were older, they gave more weight to each of these factors. Surprisingly, 79% felt that their good health was owing to "no particular reason." (Table 7.)

This study is a good beginning for future research regarding dietary factors and Alzheimer's disease. In our next phase we intend to direct a similar survey towards the care-givers of patients *with* Alzheimer's disease.

## Conclusion: Replace Aluminum with Magnesium

The debate for or against the role of aluminum in Alzheimer's disease will continue long after the publication of this book. The strongest evidence that aluminum intake and Alzheimer's disease are causally related is epidemiological; people who drink water with high concentrations of aluminum are 50 percent more likely to develop Alzheimer's disease than those whose water is aluminum free. At greatest risk, according to this study, were adults younger than age 65 (Martyn, et al., 1989). The study published here for the first time, indicates that people over 60 years of age who do *not* exhibit symptoms of Alzheimer's disease tend to ingest foods containing nutrients known to retard the bioavailability (i.e., absorption) of aluminum and to take vitamins known to protect memory and other brain functions.

Is there anything wrong with recommending low aluminum intake? It is a neurotoxic metal of *no* known use in the human body and is implicated in several disease states (see Chapter 4). There is no need to continue using aluminum in antacids, analgesics and other medications. Magnesium, already used by several manufacturers, is an equally fine carrying agent, it has all the added benefit of contributing to cardiovascular health. Prior to the 20th century, aluminum was not used in any foods or pharmaceuticals. It is no longer necessary to debate whether aluminum is the "cause or consequence" of Alzheimer's disease. That this metal is found in elevated concentrations in regions of the brain of Alzheimer's patients is reason enough to curtail its intake from *all* sources, including cookware.

We certainly do not have to lose our minds while the debate continues. Whatever the next chapter on aluminum and Alzheimer's disease may prove to be, such an environmental toxin is always preferably avoided. Given the effect of Alzheimer's on much of the aging population and the great costs, human and medical, aluminum reduction is one of our most sensible health investments.

**TABLE 1.** Nutrients from Foods

| | 3 or more times/week % | 1 or more times/week % | Total % |
|---|---|---|---|
| Choline | 12 | 16 | 28 |
| Vitamin B-12 | 19 | 30 | 49 |
| Niacin | 18 | 28 | 46 |
| Folic Acid | 21 | 25 | 46 |
| Iron | 7 | 7 | 14 |

**TABLE 2.** Alcoholic Beverages

| | 3 or more times/week % | 1 or more times/week % | Total % |
|---|---|---|---|
| Beer | 0 | 1 | 1 |
| Wine | 15 | 11 | 26 |
| Hard Liquor | 7 | 6 | 13 |
| More than one type of alcohol | 6 | 4 | 10 |
| TOTAL | 28 | 22 | 50 |

**TABLE 3.** Supplemental Vitamin Intake

| | Average Years Taken | Percentage Who Take |
|---|---|---|
| VITAMINS | | |
| Multi-vitamins | 17 | 49 |
| Vitamin A | 11 | 2 |
| Vitamin B | 16 | 21 |
| Vitamin C | 15 | 42 |
| Vitamin E | 10 | 10 |
| MINERALS | | |
| Calcium | 10 | 5 |
| Cod Liver Oil | 20 | 5 |
| Iron | 18 | 1 |
| Lecithin | 13 | 1 |
| Multi-minerals | 2 | 1 |
| Niacin | 14 | 1 |
| Zinc | 10 | 9 |

**TABLE 4.** Medications Containing Aluminum

| | Average Years Taken | Percentage Who Take |
|---|---|---|
| Antacids | 8 | 29 |
| Buffered Aspirin | 11 | 27 |
| Antidiarrheals | 9 | 3 |
| Ulcer Medicine | 5 | 7 |

**TABLE 5.** Caffeinated Beverages

| | 3 or more times/week % | 1 or more times/week % | Total % |
|---|---|---|---|
| Tea, coffee, cocoa, canned cola | 64 | 15 | 79 |

**TABLE 6.** Foods Containing Aluminum

| | 3 or more times/week % | 1 or more times/week % | Total % |
|---|---|---|---|
| Cake, flour, dough | 3 | 13 | 16 |
| Cheese | 32 | 34 | 66 |
| TOTAL | 35 | 47 | 82 |

**TABLE 7.** Self-Described Health Factors

| | GOOD HEALTH AGE | | | |
|---|---|---|---|---|
| | 68-69 | 78-79 | 80-92 | TOTAL |
| Diet | 9 | 14 | 26 | 49 |
| Exercise | 2 | 5 | 5 | 12 |
| Diet & Exercise | 4 | 10 | 13 | 27 |
| Vitamins | 0 | 1 | 2 | 3 |
| Genetics | 2 | 3 | 5 | 10 |
| Genetics, diet & exercise | 0 | 3 | 3 | 6 |
| Rest, diet | | 1 | | 1 |
| Rest, diet, exs. | | 2 | | 2 |
| No reason | 12 | 20 | 47 | 79 |
| Other than above[19] | | | | 12 |
| POOR HEALTH | | | | |
| No Reasons | | | | 14 |
| "Other" (smoking, stress, loneliness, diet) | | | | 4 |
| Respondents that did not answer these questions | | | | 2 |
| | | | TOTAL | 227 |

19 Other reasons for good health included common sense, cleanliness, sense of humor, moderation, enjoying life, keeping active, home cooking, not smoking or drinking alcohol, no-TV, travel, faith, and long marriages.

## Additional References[20]

______, Jan., 1989. Ad Hoc Working Group on Nerve Growth Factor and Alzheimer's Disease: Potential use of nerve growth factor to treat Alzheimer's disease. *Science.*

______, Feb., 1989. Aluminum and Alzheimer's disease (letter). *Lancet,* 1 (8632):267-9.

Axelson, O., M. Hane, C. Hogstedt, 1976. A case-referrent study on neuropsychiatric disorders among workers exposed to solvents. *Scan J Work Environ Health* 2:14-20.

Birchall, J.D., J.S. Chappell, 1989. The chemistry of aluminum and silicon in relation to Alzheimer's Disease. *Clin Chem 34/2, 265-267.*

Coriat, A. M., R. D. Gillard. 1986 *Nature* 321, 570.

Cox, N. H., C. Moss, A. Forsyth. July 2, 1988. Cutaneous reactions to aluminum in vaccines: an avoidable problem. *Lancet,* p. 43.

Coyle, J. T., D. L. Price, M. R. Delong. 1983. Alzheimer's disease: a disorder or cortical cholinergic innervation. *Science 219:1184-1190.*

20 These references include the latest information available and supplement the bibliography included in the hardcover edition of this book.

Crapper, D. R., S. S. Krisnan, S. Quittkat. 1976. Aluminum, Neurofibrillary degeneration and Alzheimer's disease. *Braini 99: 67-80.*

English, D., D. Cohen. 1985. A case-control study of maternal age in Alzheimer's disease. *J Am Geriatr Soc 33: 167-169.*

Flaten, T. P., M. Odegard. Nov./Dec., 1988. Tea, aluminum and Alzheimer's disease (letter). *Food and Chemical Toxicology 26 (11-12):959-60.*

Fleming, L. W., A. Prescott, W. K. Steward, R. W. Cargill. Feb. 25, 1989. Bioavailability of aluminum (letter). *Lancet 1 (8635):433.*

French, L. R., L. M. Shuman, J. A. Mortimer, et al. April, 1989. A case-control study of dementia of the Alzheimer type. *Am J Epidemiol 121:414-421.*

Grundke-Igbal, I., et al. April, 1989. Amyloid protein and neurofibrillary tangles coexist in the same neuron in Alzheimer disease. *Proc Natl Acad Sci, USA, Vol 86*, pp. 2853-2857.

Hefti, F., W. J. Weiner. 1986. Nerve growth factor and Alzheimer's disease. *Annals of Neurology, 20:275-281.*

Henderson, A. S. 1988. The risk factors for Alzheimer's disease: a review and a hypothesis. *Acta psychiat. scand. Art 1039.*

Henderson, V. W., C. E. Finch. March, 1989. The neurobiology of Alzheimer's disease. *Journal of Neurosurgery, 70(3):335-53.*

Hughes, J. T. March 4, 1989. Aluminum encephalopathy and Alzheimer's disease. *Lancet, 1(8636):490-1.*

Krishnam, S. S., D. R. McLachlan, B. Krishnan, S. S. Fenton, J. E. Harrison. April, 1988. Aluminum toxicity to the brain. *Sci Total Environ, 71(1):59-64.*

Kushnir, S. L., J. T. Ratner, P. A. Gregoire. May, 1987. Multiple Nutrients in the Treatment of Alzheimer's disease. *Amer Geriatrics Soc J (35)5:476-477.*

Levi-Montalcini, R. 1987. The nerve growth factor 35 years later. *Science 273:1154-1162.*

Lukiw, W. J., T. P. Kruck, D. R. McLachlan. 1987. Alterations in human linker histone-DNA binding in the presence of aluminum salts in vitro and in Alzheimer's disease. *Neurotoxicology 8(2):291-301.*

Martyn, C. N., D. J. Barker, C. Osmond, E. C. Harris, J. A. Edwardson, R. F. Lacey. January, 1989. Geographical relation between Alzheimer's disease and aluminum in drinking water. *Lancet 1(8629):59-62.*

McLachlan, D. R., M. F. Van Berkum. 1986. Aluminum: a roll in degenerative brain disease associated with neurofibrillary degeneration. *Prog Brain Res, 70:399-410.*

McLachlan, D. R. Nov./Dec., 1986. Aluminum and Alzheimer's disease. *Neurobiol Aging 7(6):525-32.*

Rocca, W. A. 1986. A case control study showing "a significant association with the use of aluminum-containing anti-perspirants." *Am Jour Epid, 126-754.*

Rocca, W. A., L. A. Amducci, B. S. Schoenberg. 1986. Epidemiology of clinically diagnosed Alzheimer's disease. *Ann Neurol 19:415-424.*

Schoenberg, B. S. 1981. Methodological approaches to the epidemiologic study of dementia. In Mortimer, J. A., L. M. Schuman (eds): The Epiodemiology of Dementia. New York, *Oxford Univ Press* pp. 117-131.

Schroeder, H. A. 1973. The Trace Elements and Man, Some Positive and Negative Aspects. *The Devin-Adair Company,* Old Greenwich CT.

Tennakone, K., S. Wickramanayake. January, 1987. Aluminum leaking from cooking utensils. *Nature,* Vol 325.

Youdim, M. B. H. January, 1988. Iron in the brain: implications for Parkinson's and Alzheimer's diseases. *Mt. Sinai J of Med,* Vol 55, No. 1.

# Selected Bibliography[21]


Abalan, F. 1984. Alzheimer's disease and malnutrition: A new etiological hypothesis. *Medical Hypotheses*, 15: 385-93.

______2/5/86. Personal communication.

Bjorksten, J., Ph.D. 1980. The Crosslinkage theory of aging as a predictive indicator. *Rejuvenation VIII*, 3: 59-66.

______1983. The conversion of euchromatin to heterochromatin (An aspect of Alzheimer's disease). *Rejuvenation XI*, 4: 101-10.

Brun, A., and N. Dictor, 1981. Senile plaques and tangles in dialysis dementia. *Acta. Path. Mcrobiol. Scand.* Sect. A, 89: 193-98.

Cam, J. M., V. A. Luck, J. B. Eastwood and H. E. deWardener. 1976. The effects of aluminum hydroxide orally on calcium, phosphorus and aluminum metabolism in normal subjects. *Clin. Sci. Mol. Med.*, 51: 407-19.

Candy, J. M., J. A. Edwardson. February 15, 1986. Aluminosilicates and senile plaque formation in Alzheimer's disease. *Lancet*, 1: 354.


21 While the references are intended to guide the interested reader to original sources, a complete list is not provided. Those studies relating to nutrition and aluminum, the main theses of this book, are provided.

Cantor, D. S., et al. 1986. A report on phosphatidylcholine therapy in a Down's syndrome child. *Psychological Reports*, 58: 207-17.

Casdorph, R. H., M.D., Ph.D. 1981. EDTA chelation therapy II, efficacy in brain disorders. *J. Hol. Med., 3, (2):* Fall/Winter.

Cathcart, III, Robert F. 1985. Vitamin C: The nontoxic, nonrate-limited, antioxidant free radical scavenger. *Medical Hypotheses*, 18: 61-77.

Chen, K. M., Y. Yase. 1983. Amyotrophic lateral sclerosis in Asia and Oceania. Taiwan: Shyan-Fu Chou, National Taiwan University.

Clarkson, E. M., V. A. Luck, W. V. Hynson, R. R. Bailey, J. B. Eastwood, J. S. Clements, J. L. H. O'Riordan, and H. E. Wardner. 1972. The effects of aluminum hydroxide on calcium, phosphorus and aluminum balances, the serum parathyroid hormone concentration and the aluminum content of bone in patients with chronic renal failure. *Clin. Sci., 43:* 519-31.

Coburn, J. W., A. S. Brickman, D. J. Sherrard, F. R. Singer, E. G. C. Wong, D. J. Baylink and A. W. Norman. 1977. Use of 1,25(OH)2-vitamin D3 to separate "types" of renal osteodystrophy. *Proc. EDTA., 14*: 442-50.

Cochran, M., M. M. Platts, P. J. Moorhead, and A. Buxton. 1981. Spontaneous hypercalcemia in maintenance dialysis patients: An association with atypical osteomalacia and fractures. *Mineral and Electrolyte Metab., 5*: 280-86.

Cooke, N., S. Teitelbaum, and L. V. Avioli. 1978. Antacid-induced osteomalacia and nephrolithiasis. *Arc. Inter. Med., 138:* 1007-9.

Cooper, G. P., G. L. Krueger, and E. M. Widner. May 21, 1981. Neurotoxicity of Aluminum. Prepared for The Aluminum Association. Dept. of Environmental Health, College of Medicine, Univ. of Cincinnati, Ohio.

Cournot-Witmer, G., J. Zingraff, R. Bourdon, T. Drueke, and S. Balsan. 1979. Aluminum and dialysis bone disease. *Lancet, 2:* 795-96.

Cournot-Witmer, G., J. Zingraff, J. J. Plachot, F. Escaig, R. Lefevre, P. Boumati, A. Bourdeau, M. Garabedian, P. Galle, R. Boudon, T. Drueke, and S. Balsan. 1981. Aluminum localization in bone from hemodialyzed patients: Relationship to matrix mineralization. *Kidney Internal, 20*: 375-85.

Cox, G. J., H. L. Dodds, H. B. Wigman, and F. J. Murphy. 1931. The effects of high doses of aluminum and iron phosphorus metabolism. *J. Biol. Chem., 92*: 11-12.

Cranton, E. 1985. *Bypassing Bypass.* Stein and Day, Publishers, Briarcliff Manor, New York.

Crapper, D. R. 1974. Dementia: Recent observation on Alzheimer's disease and experimental aluminum encephalopathy. In: Seeman, P. M. and G. M. Brown, (eds). *Frontiers of Neurology and Neuroscience Research.* University of Toronto Press, Toronto. 97-111.

Crapper, D. R. and Dalton, A. J. 1973. Alterations in short-term retention, conditioned avoidance response acquisition and motivation following aluminum induced neurofibrillary degeneration. *Physiol and Behav., 10*: 925-33.

Crapper, D. R. and U. De Boni. 1977. Aluminum and the genetic apparatus in Alzheimer's disease. In: Nandy, K. and I.

Sherwin, (eds). *The Aging Brain and Senile Dementia*. Plenum Press, New York and London, 229-46.

Crapper McLachlan, D. R. and U. De Boni. 1980. Aluminum in human brain disease—An overview. *Neurotoxicology 1*: 3-16.

Crapper, D. R. S. S. Krishnan, and S. Quittak. 1976. Aluminum, neurofibrillary degeneration and Alzheimer's disease. *Brain*, 99: 67-80.

Crapper McLachlan, D. R., S. S. Krishnan, S. Quittkat, and U. De Boni. 1980. Brain aluminum in Alzheimer's disease: Influence of sample size and case selection. *Neurotoxicology, 1*: 25-32.

Crapper, D. R., S. Quittake, S. S. Krishnan, A. J. Dalton, and U. De Boni. 1980. Intranuclear aluminum content in Alzheimer's disease, dialysis encephalopathy, and experimental aluminum encephalopathy. *Acta Neuropath. (Berl) 50*: 19-24.

Crapper, D. R. and G. Tomko. 1975. Neuronal correlates of an encephalopathy associated with aluminum neurofibrillary degeneration. *Brain Research. 97*: 253-64.

Cuisinier-Gleizes, P., A. George, C. Giullano, and H. Mathieu. 1971. Stimulation of bone resorption by phosphorus deprivation in the rat. *Israel J. Med. Sci.*, 7 (3): 355.

Dalton, A. J., S. N. Cibiri, J. G. Baker, H. S. Malik, and B. Wu. 1981. Basic life skills scale; Manual of norms and standardization. Ministry of Community and Social Services. Toronto.

Dalton, A. J. and D. R. Crapper. 1977. Down's syndrome and the brain. In: Peter Mittler (ed.). *Research to Practice in Mental Retardation*. Vol. III Biomedical Aspects. University Park Press, Baltimore. 391-400.

Dalton, A. J., D. R. Crapper, and G. R. Schlotterer. 1973. Alzheimer's disease in Down's syndrome: Visual retention deficits. *Cortex, 10*: 366-77.

Davies, P., and A. J. F. Maloney. 1976. Selective loss of central cholinergic neurons in Alzheimer's disease. *Lancet,* 2: 1403.

Davis, K. L., et al 1979. Enhancement of memory by physostigmines. *N. Engl. J. Med., 301*: 946.

Dayan, A. P. and M. J. Ball. 1973. Histiometric observations of the metabolism of tangle bearing neurons. *J. Neurol. Sci., 19*: 433-36.

De Boni, U., A. Otvos, J. W. Scott, and Crapper, D. R. 1976. Neurofibrillary degeneration induced by systemic aluminum. *Acta. Neuropath. (Berl) 35*: 285-94.

De Boni, U., J. W. Scott, and D. R. Crapper. 1974. Intracellular aluminum binding; a histochemical study. *Histochem., 40*: 31-37.

Dent, C. E. and C. S. Winter. 1974. Osteomalacia due to phosphate depletion from excessive aluminum hydroxide ingestion. *Br. Med. J., 23*: 551-52.

Drueke, T. 1980. Dialysis osteomalacia and aluminum intoxication, *Nephron, 26*: 207-10.

Edwardson, James. 1986. Aluminosilicates at the core of senile plaques. *Lancet, 1*: 354.

Elliott, H. L. and A. I. MacDougall. 1978. Aluminum studies in dialysis encephalopathy. *Proc. Eur. Dial. Trans. Assoc., 15*: 157-63.

___1980. Dialysis encephalopathy—evidence implicating aluminum. *Dialysis and Transplantation, 9 (11):* 1027-30.

Elliott, H. L., A. I. MacDougall, and G. S. Fell. 1978a. Aluminum toxicity syndrome. *Lancet*, 1: 1203.

Elliot, H. L., A. I. MacDougall, G. S. Fell, and P. H. E, Gardiner. 1978b. Plasmapheresis, aluminum and dialysis dementia. *Lancet*, 2: 1255.

Ellis, H. A., J. H. McCarthy, and J. Herrington. 1979. Bone aluminum in haemodialysed patients and in rats injected with aluminum chloride: Relationship to impaired bone mineralisation. *J. Clin. Pathol., 32*: 832-44.

Ellis, H. A., A. M. Pierides, T. G. Feest, M. K. Ward, and D. N. S. Kerr, 1977. Histopathology of renal osteodystrophy with particular reference to the effects of 1—hydroxyvitamin D3 in patients treated by long-term hemodialysis. *Clin. Endocrinology, 7 (Suppl)*: 31S-38S.

Epstein, Seymour G. 1984. Aluminum and health: A discussion of Alzheimer's disease. The Aluminum Assoc. Washington, D.C.

Etienne, P., et al. 1978. Clinical effects of choline in Alzheimer's disease. *Lancet, 1*: 508-9.

Fauley, G. B., S. Freeman, A. C. Ivy, A. J. Atkinson, and H. S. Wigodsky. 1941. Aluminum phosphate in the therapy of peptic ulcer: Effects of aluminum hydroxide on phosphate absorption. *Arch. Intern. Med., 67*: 63-78.

Feinroth M., M. V. Feinroth, E. A. Friedman, and G. M. Berlyne. 1980. Effect of parathyroid hormone and acute renal failure on aluminum absorption in rat everted gut sacs. *Clin. Res., 28*: 656 A.

Felsenfeld, A. J., J. M. Harrelson, R. A. Gutman, S. A. Wells, and M. K. Drezner. 1982. Osteomalacia after parathyroidectomy in patients with uremia. *Ann. Intern. Med., 96:* 34-39.

Ferry, Georgina. February 27, 1986. Aluminosilicates at the centre of dementia. *New Scientist,* 23.

Firschein, H. E. 1969. Phosphate as a regulator of bone collagen and mineral resorption. *Fed. Amer. Soc. Exp. Biol. Proc., 28:* 374. Abstr. #656.

Fishman, M., M.D., H. Merskey, M.D., E. Helmes, J. McCready, E. H. Colhoun, and B. J. Rylett. October 1981. Double blind study of lecithin in patients with Alzheimer's disease. *Can. J. Psychiatry, 26.*

Flendrig, J. A., H. Kruis, and H. A. Das. 1976. Aluminum intoxication: The cause of dialysis dementia? *Proc. Eur. Dial. Transplant. Assoc., 13:* 355-64.

Garcia-Bunuel, L., D. C. Elliot, and N. K. Bank. 1980. Apneic spells in progressive dialysis encephalopathy. *Archs. Neurol. (Chicago),* 37: 594-96.

Giudicelli, C. P. 1982. Toxicite de Taluminium pour l'hepatocyte. Localisation ultrastructurale et micro-analyse des depots. *La Nouvelle Presse Medicale, 11 (15):* 1123-25.

Goldsmith, Marsha F. April 13, 1984. Attempts to vanquish Alzheimer's disease intensify, take new paths. *JAMA, 251 (14):*1805-40.

Goodman, F. R. and G. B. Weiss. 1971a. Dissociation by lanthanum of smooth muscle responses to potassium and acetylcholine. *Amer. J. Physiol., 220:* 759-66.

______1971b. Effects of lanthanum on 45 Ca movements and on contractions induced by norepinephrine, histamine and potassium in vascular smooth muscle. *J. Pharmacol. Exptl. Therap., 177:* 415-25.

Gorsky, J. E., A. A. Dietz, H. Spencer, and D. Osis. 1979. Metabolic balance of aluminum studied in six men. *Clin. Chem., 25, (10):* 1739-43.

Hava, M. and A. Hurwitz. 1973. The relaxing effect of aluminum and lanthanum on rat and human gastric smooth muscle in vitro. *Eur. J. Pharmacol., 22:* 156-61.

Henderson, D. 1982. *Cookware as a source of additives.* FDA Consumer. Dept. of Health & Human Services. HHS Publication No. (FDA) 82-2162.

Hodsman, A. B., D. J. Sherrard, A. C. Alfrey, S. Ott, A. S. Brickman, N. L. Miller, N. A. Maloney, and J. W. Coburn. 1982. Bone aluminum and histomorphometric features of renal osteodystrophy. *J. Clin. Endocrinology and Metab., 54 (3):* 539-46.

Hodsman, A. B., D. J. Sherrard, E. G. C. Wong, A. S. Brickman, D. B. Lee, A. C. Alfrey, F. R. Singer, A. W. Norman, and J. W. Coburn. 1981. Vitamin D resistant osteomalacia in hemodialysis patients lacking secondary hyperparathyroidism. *Ann. Intern. Med., 94:* 629-37.

Hoffer, A., M. Walker. 1980. *Nutrients to Age Without Senility.* Connecticut: Keats Publishing Company.

Huber, C. T. and E. Frieden. 1970. The inhibition of ferroxidase by trivalent and other metal ions, *J. Biol. Chem., 245:* 3979-84.

Hurwitz, A. 1971. The effects of antacids on gastrointestinal drug absorption. II. Effect of sulfadiazine and quinine. *J. Pharmacol. Exptl. Therap.,* 179: 485-89.

Hurwitz, A. and M. B. Sheehan. 1971. The effects of antacids on the absorption of orally administered pentobarbitol in the rat. *J. Pharmacol. Exptl. Therap., 179:* 124-31.

Insogna, K. L., D. R. Bordley, J. F. Caro, and D. H. Lockwood. 1980. Osteomalacia and weakness from excessive antacid ingestion. *JAMA., 244:* 2544-46.

Ishii, T. 1966. Distribution of Alzheimer's neurofibrillary changes in the brain stem and hypothalamus of senile dementia. *Actaw neuropath. (Berl) 6:* 181-87.

Jeejeebhoy, K. N. 1982. Therapeutique dietetique et nutrition parenterale. In Harrison, T. R., *Principes de medecine interne.* Flammarion Ed., (3rd. ed.), Paris.

Jordan, J. W. 1961. Pulmonary fibrosis in a worker using aluminum power. *Birt. J. Ind. Med., 18:* 21.

Jowsey, J., W. J. Johnson, D. R. Taves, and P. H. Kelly. 1972. Effects of dialysate calcium and fluoride on bone disease during hemodialyses. *J. Lab. Clin. Med., 79:* 204-14.

Kaehny, W. D., A. C. Alfrey, R. E. Holman, and W. J. Shorr. 1977a. Aluminum transfer during hemodialysis. *Kidney International, 12:* 361-65.

Kaehny, W. D., A. P. Hegg, and A. C. Alfrey. 1977b. Gastrointestinal absorption of aluminum from aluminum containing antacids. *N. Engl. J. Med., 296:* 1389-91.

Karlil, S. J. 1979. Aluminum interactions with DNA and other poynucleotides. Ph.D. thesis, University of Toronto.

Katz, A. M. 1970. Contractile proteins of the heart. *Physiol., Rev. 50 (1): 63-158.*

Katzman, R., M.D. April 1986, Alzheimer's Disease. *N. Engl. J. Med., 314 (15):964-73.*

Kehow, R. A., J. Cholak, and R. V. Storey. 1940. Spectrochemical study of the normal ranges of concentration of certain trace metals in biological materials. *J. Nutrition, 19:* 579-92.

Kerr, D. N. S. 1981. Renal osteomalacia. In: Proceedings of the Eighth International Congress of Nephrology. Zurukzoglu, W., M. Papadimitriou, M. Pyrpasopoulos, M. Sion, and C. Zamboulis, eds. Bassle: Krager, 221-28.

King, R. G. 1984. Do raised brain aluminum levels in Alzheimer's dementia contribute to cholinergic neuronal deficits? Department of Pharmacology, Monash University, Australia. *Medical Hypotheses 14:* 301-6.

King, S. W., M. R. Wills, and J. Savory. 1979. Serum binding of aluminum. *Res. Commun. Chem. Pathol. Pharmacol., 26:* 161-69.

Kirsner, J. B. 1943. Effect of calcium carbonate, aluminum phosphate, and aluminum hydroxide on mineral excretion in man. *J. Clin. Invest, 22:* 47-52.

Klein, G. L., C. M. Targoff, M. E. Ament, D. J. Sherrard, R. Bluestone, J. H. Young, A. W. Norman, and J. W. Coburn. 1980. Bone disease associated with total parenteral nutrition. *Lancet, 2:* 1041-44.

Kovalchik, M. T., W. D. Kaehny, A. P. Hegg, F. T. Jackson, and A. C. Alfrey. 1978. Aluminum kinetics during hemodialysis. *J. Lab. Clin. Med., 92, (5):* 712-20.

Kraut, J. A., J. H. Shinaberger, F. R. Singer, D. J. Sherrard, J. Saxton, J. H. Miller, K. Kurokawa, and J. W. Coburn. 1983. Parathyroid gland responsiveness to acute hypocalcemia in dialysis osteomalacia. *Kidney Int., 23:* 725-30.

Lai, J. C. K., J. F. Guest, T. K. C. Leung, L. Lim, and A. N. Davison. 1980. The effects of cadmium, manganese and aluminum on sodium-potassium-activated and magnesium-activated adenosine triphosphatase activity and choline uptake in rat brain synaptosomes. *Biochem. Pharma., 29:* 141-46.

Lehmann, J., S. Persson, J. Walinder, and L. Wallin. 1981. Tryptophan malabsorption in dementia. Improvement in certain cases after tryptophan therapy as indicated by mental behaviour and blood analysis. A Pilot Study. *Acta psychiat. Scand., 64:* 123-31.

Lehninger, A. L. 1981. Vitamines et coenzymes. In *Bichimie.* Flammarion Ed. 2nd. Ed., Paris, p. 331.

Levy, Raymond. 1985. Rational drug treatment of dementia? *Brit Med. J., 291: 139.*

Lieberherr, M., B. Grosse, G. Cournot-Witmer, C. L. Thil, and Balsan. 1982. In vitro effects of aluminum on bone phosphatases: A possible interaction with PTH and vitamin D3 metabolites, *Calcif. Tissue Int., 34:* 280-84.

Lione, A. 1983. The prophylactic reduction of aluminum intake. *Fd. Chem. Toxic, 21 (1):* 103-9.

______1985A. Aluminum intake from non-prescription drugs and sucralfate. *Gen. Pharmac., 16 (3):* 223-28.

______Sept./Oct. 1985B. The reduction of aluminum intake in patients with Alzheimer's disease, *J. Environmental Path., Tox. & Onc., 6: 2l.*

Liss, L., et al. 1976. Facilitation of Alzheimer's dementia by exogenous factors. *Jour Neuropathol. Exp. Neurol.,* 35:372, abstract no. 145.

Litman, A. 1967. Reactive and nonreactive aluminum hydroxide gels: Dose-response relationships in vivo. *Gastroenterology, 52: 948-51.*

Little, Adrienne, et al. 1985. A double-blind, placebo-controlled trial of high-dose lecithin in Alzheimer's disease. *Jour. Neurology, Neurosurgery, and Psychiatry, 48:* 736-42.

Lotz, M., E. Zisman, and F. C. Bartter. 1968. Evidence for a phosphorous-depletion syndrome in man. *N. Engl. J. Med.* 278: 409-15.

Mann, D., D. Neary, P. Yates, J. Lincoln, J. Snowden, and P. Stanworth. 1981. Alterations in protein synthetic capability of nerve cells in Alzheimer's disease. *J. Neurol. Neurosurg. Psych., 44:* 97-102.

Mann, D. M. A. and K. G. A. Sinclair, 1978. The quantitative assessment of lipofusine pigment, cytoplasmic RNA and nucleolar volume in senile dementia. *Neuropath. Applied Neurobiol., 4:* 129-35.

Matsumoto, H., E. Hirasaw, and E. Takahashi. 1976. Localization of aluminum in tea leaves. *Plant and Cell Physiol., 17:* 627-31.

Mayor, G. H., J. Keiser, D. Makdani, and P. K. Ku. 1977. Aluminum absorption and distribution: Effect of parathyroid hormone. *Science, 197:* 1187-89.

Mayor, G. H., T. O. Lohr, T. V. Sanchez, and M. A. Burnatowska-Hledin. Sept./Oct. 1985. Aluminum metabolism and toxicity in renal failure: A review, *J. Envir., Path., Tox., & Onc., 6*: 43.

Mayor, G. H., S. M. Sprague, M. R. Hourani and T. V. Sanchez. 1980. Parathyroid hormone-medicated aluminum deposition and egress in the rat. *Kidney Int., 17*: 40-44.

McDermott, J. R., A. I. K. Smith, K. Igbal, and H. M. Wisniewski. 1977. Aluminum and Alzheimer's disease. *Lancet, 2*: 710-11.

McLaughlin, A. I. G., G. Kazontzis, E. King, D. Teare, J. J. Porter, and R. Owen. 1962. Pulmonary fibrosis and encephalopathy associated with the inhalation of aluminum dust. *Brit. J. Med. 19*: 253.

Menkes, Marilyn S., et al. November 13, 1986. Serum beta-carotene, vitamins A and E, selenium, and the risk of lung cancer. *N. Engl. J. Med., 315 (20)*: 1250-54.

Meredith, P. A., H. L. Elliot, B. C. Campbell, and M. R. Moore. 1979. Changes in serum aluminum, blood zinc, blood lead, and erythrocyte delta-aminolaevulinic acid dehydratase activity during haemodialysis. *Toxicol. Lett., 4*: 419-24.

Mikelens, P., and W. Levinson. 1978. Nucleic acid binding by tetracycline-metal ion complexes. *Bioinorganic Chemistry, 9*: 421-29.

Miller, C. A. and E. M. Levine. 1974. Effect of aluminum gels on cultured neuroblastoma cells. *J. Neurochem., 22*: 751-58.

Mitchell, J. 1959. Pulmonary Fibrosis in an aluminum worker. *Brit. J. Ind. Med.,16*: 123.

Mitchell, J., et al. 1961. Pulmonary fibrosis in workers exposed to finely powdered aluminum. *Brit. J. Ind. Med., 18*: 10.

Morrissey, J., M. G. Mayor, and E. Slatopolsky. 1983. Suppression of parathyroid hormone secretion by aluminum. *Kidney Int., 23*: 699-704.

O'Hare, J. A. and D. J. Murnaghan. 1982. Reversal of aluminum induced hemodialysis anemia by a low-aluminum dialysate. *N. Engl. J. Med., 306*: 654-56.

Ott, S. M., N. A. Maloney, A. C. Alfrey, J. W. Coburn, and D. J. Sherrard. 1981. Prevalence of aluminum (Al) in bone from uremic patients. American Soc. of Nephrology, 14th. Annual Meeting, Abstract No. 43.

Ott, S. M., N. A. Maloney, G. L. Klein, A. C. Alfrey, M. E. Ament, J. W. Coburn, and D. J. Sherrard. 1983. Aluminum is associated with low bone formation in patients receiving chronic parenteral nutrition. *Ann. Int. Med., 98*: 910-14.

Parkinson, I. S., M. K. Ward, T. G. Feest, R. W. P. Fawcett, and D. N. S. Kerr. 1979. Fracturing dialysis osteodystrophy and dialysis encephalopathy: An epidemiological survey. *Lancet, 1*: 406-9.

Parsons, V., C. Davies, C. Goode, C. Ogg, and J. Siddiqui. 1971. Aluminum in bone from patients with renal failure. *Br. Med. J., 4*: 273-75.

Perl, D. P. and A. R. Brody. 1979. Detection of focal accumulations of aluminum (Al) and silicon (Si) within neurofibrillary tangle bearing neurons of Alzheimer's disease. *J. Neuropath. 1 Exp. Neurol., 38, Abstract 102*: 335.

Perl, D. P., D. Gajdusek, R. Garruto, R. Yanagrhara, and C. Gibbs. 1982. Intraneuronal aluminum accumulation in amyotrophic lateral sclerosis and Parkinsonism-dementia of Guam. *Science, 217*: 1053-55.

Peruzza, Marino, M.D. and Maurizio DeJacobis, M.D. July/August 1986. A double-blind placebo controlled evaluation of the efficacy and safety of vinpocetine in the treatment of patients with chronic vascular or degenerative senile cerebral dysfunction. *Advances In Therapy., 3 (4).*

Petit, T. L., G. B. Biederman, and P. A. McMullen. 1980. Neurofibrillary degeneration, dendritic dying back and learning-memory deficits following aluminum administration: Implications for brain aging. *Exper. Neurol., 67*: 152-62.

Platts, M. M., G. C. Goode, and J. S. Hislop. 1977. Composition of the domestic water supply and the incidence of fractures and encephalopathy in patients on home dialysis. *Br. Med. J., 2:* 657-60.

Provone, P., N. H. Bell, and F. C. Bartter. 1961. Production of hypercalaciuria by phosphorous deprivation on a low calcium intake: A new clinical test for hyperparathyroidism. *Metabolism, 10*: 364-71.

Rich, C., J. Ennsinck, and P. Ivanovich. 1964. The effects of sodium flouride and calcium metabolism of subjects with metabolic bone diseases. *J. Clin. Invest., 43*: 545-56.

Robertson, J. A., A. J. Felsenfeld, C. C. Haygood, P. Wilson, C. Clarke, and F. Llach. 1983. Animal model of aluminum-induced osteomalacia: Role of chronic renal failure. Kidney *Internat., 23*: 327-35.

Seller, R. H. 1971. The role of magnesium in digitalis toxicity. *Amer. Heart J., 82*: 551-56.

Shaner, C. G. and A. R. Riddell. 1947. Lung changes associated with the D. R. Manufacture of aluminum abrasives. *J. Ind. Hgg. Toxicol., 29*: 113.

Shields, H. M. 1978. Rapid fall of serum phosphorus secondary to antacid therapy. *Gastroenterology, 75*: 1137-41.

Shike, M., J. E. Harrison, W. C. Sturtridge, M. D. Sturtridge, C. S. Tam, P. E. Bobechko, G. Jones, T. M. Murray, and K. N. Jeejeebhoy. 1980. Metabolic bone disease in patients receiving long-term total parenteral nutrition. *Ann. Int. Med., 92:* 343-50.

Shiraki, H. and Y. Yase. 1975. Amyotrophic Lateral Sclerosis in Japan. In: Vinken P. J. and G. W. Bruyn, eds. *Handbook of Clinical Neurology*, vol. 22. New York: Elsevier: 353-419.

Shore, D., S. W. King, W. Kaye, E. F. Torrey, H. J. Winfrey, S. G. Potkin, D. R. Winberger, J. Savory, M. R. Willis, and R. J. Wyatt. 1980. Serum and cerebrospinal fluid aluminum and circulating parathyroid hormone in primary degenerative (senile) dementia. *Neurotoxicology, 1 (4):* 55-65.

Shore, D., M. Stuart, G. Sprague, G. H. Mayor, C. Moreno, P. S. Apostoles, and R. J. Wyatt. Sept./Oct. 1985. Aluminum-Floride Complexes: Preclinical Studies. *J. Envir., Path., Tox., & Onc., 6*: 9.

Shorr, E. and A. C. Carter. 1950. Aluminum gels in the management of renal phosphatic calculi. *JAMA, 144*: 1543-56.

Short, A. I. K., R. J. Winney, and J. S. Robson. 1980. Reversible microcytic hypochromic anaemia in dialysis patients due to aluminum intoxication. *Proc. Eur. Dial. Trans. Assoc., 17*: 226-33.

Signoret, J. L., et al. 1978. Influence of choline on amnesia in early Alzheimer's disease. *Lancet, 2*: 837.

Sorenson, J. R. J., R. Campbell, L. B. Tepper, and R. D. Lingg. 1974. Aluminum in the environment and human health. *Environmental Health Perspectives, 8*: 3-95.

Spencer, H., L. Kramer, C. Norris, and D. Osis. 1982. Effect of small doses of aluminum-containing antacids on calcium and phosphorus metabolism. *Amer. J. Nutr., 36*: 32-40.

Spencer, H., L. Kramer, C. Norris, D. Osis, and E. Wiatroski, 1980a. Effect of aluminum on fluoride and calcium metabolism in man. In: *Trace Substances in Environmental Health XIV*. D. D. Hemphill (ed.), Univ. of Missouri, Columbia.

Spencer, H., L. Kramer, C. Norris, and E. Wiatroski, 1980b. Effect of aluminum hydroxide on fluoride metabolism. *Clinical Pharmacology and Therapeutics, 28 (4):* 529-35.

Spencer, H., I. Lewin, D. Osis, and J. Samachson. 1970. Studies of fluoride and calcium metabolism in patients with osteoporosis. *Am. J. Med., 49*: 814-22.

Terry, R. D. and C. Pena. 1965. Experimental production of neurofibrillary degeneration. (2) Electron microscopy, phosphatase histochemistry and electron probe analysis. *J. Neuropath. Exp. Neurol., 24*: 200-10.

Thal, L. J. M.D., P. A. Fuld, Ph.D., D. M. Masur, M.S., and S. Sharpless, Ph.D. 1983. Oral Physostigmine and Lecithin Improve Memory in Alzheimer's Disease. *Ann. Neurol. 13:*491-96.

Toda, W., J. Lux, and J. C. Van Loon. 1980. Determination of aluminum in solution from gel filtration chromatography of human serum by electrothermal atomic absorption spectroscopy. *Anal. Letters, 13 (B13):* 1105-13.

Touam, M., F. Martinez, B. Lacour, R. Bourdon, J. Zingraff, S. Di Giulio, and T. Drueke. 1983. Aluminum-induced, reversible microcyric anemia in chronic renal failure: clinical and experimental studies. *Clin. Nephrology, 19*: 295-98.

Trapp, G. A. 1983. Plasma aluminum is bound to transferrin. *Life Sci., 33*: 311-16.

______Sept./Oct. 1985. Aluminum binding to organic acids and plasma proteins: Implications for dialysis encephalopathy. 1985. *J. Envir., Path., Tox., & Onc., 6 (15).*

Trapp, G. A., G. D. Miner, R. L. Zimmerman, A. R. Mastri, and L. L. Heston. 1978. Aluminum levels in brain in Alzheimer's disease. *Biol. Psych., 13*: 709-18.

Ullmann, F. 1965. Metallbestimmungen in dosenbier. *Schweiz. Brau. Rundschau, 76 (6):* 104.

Underwood, E. J. 1977. *Trace elements in human and animal nutrition.* 4th edit. Academic Press, New York.

Varghese, Z., J. F. Moorhead, and M. R. Wills. 1973. Plasma calcium and magnesium fractions in chronic renal failure patients on maintenance haemodialysis. *Lancet, 2*: 985-88.

Verbeelen, D., J. Smeyers-Verbeke, and D. L. Massart. 1980. Aluminum (Al) containing antacids: source of high serum Al levels in patients treated with regular hemodialysis. *Toxico. Lett., 1*: 61-68.

Walker, J. A. M.D., R. A. Sherman, M.D., and R. P. Eisinger, M.D. Oct. 1985. Thrombocytopenia associated with intravenous desferrioxamine. *Amer. J. Kidney Dx., VI (4).*

Wang, H. S. In: *Aging and Dementia.* W. Smith and M. Kinsbourne (eds.). *Spectrum Press,* New York. 1-24.

Ward, M. K., T. G. Feest, H. A. Ellis, I. S. Parkinson, D. N. S. Kerr, J. Harrington, and G. L. Goode. 1978. Osteomalacic dialysis osteodystrophy: Evidence for a water-borne aetiological agent probably aluminum. *Lancet, 1*: 841-45.

Weiss, G. B. and F. R. Goodman. 1969. Effects of lanthanum on contraction, calcium distribution and Ca movements in intestinal smooth muscle, *J. Pharmacol. Exptl. Therap., 169*: 46-55.

Williams, P., R. Khanna, D. R. Crapper. 1981. Enhancement of removal of aluminum by desferrioxamine in a patient on continuous ambulatory peritoneal dialysis with dementia. *Peritoneal Dialysis Bulletin 1.*

Wills, M. R., and J. Savory. 1983. Aluminum poisoning: Dialysis encephalopathy, osteomalacia, and anaemia. *Lancet, 2:* 29-33.

Wing, A. J., C. P. Brunner, H. Brynger, C. Chatler, B. A. Donckerwolocke, H. J. Gurland, C. Jacobs, P. Kramer, and N. H. Selwood. 1980. Dialysis dementia in Europe: Report from the European dialysis and transplant association. *Lancet, 2:* 190-92.

Wisniewski, H., H. Narang, and R. Terry. 1976. Neurofibrillary tangles of paired helical filaments, *J. Neurol. Sci., 27*: 173-81.

Wisniewski, H., O. Narkiewicz, and K. Wisniewska, 1967. Topography and dynamics of neurofibrillary degeneration in aluminum encephalopathy. *ACTA Neuropath., 9*: 127-33.

Wisniewski, H. M., J. A. Sturmanm, J. A. Shek, J. W. Iqbal. Sept./Oct. 1985. Aluminum and the Central Nervous System. *J. Envir. Path., Tox., & Onc., 6 (1).*

Wolozin, B. L., A. Pruchnicki, D. W. Dickson, and P. Davies. May 1986. A neuronal antigen in the brains of Alzheimer patients. *Science, 232*: 648-50.

Wurtman, R. J. 1982. *Alzheimer's Disease: A Report of Progress in Aging*. Corking S., ed. New York: Raven Press, vol. 19, 495.

Wurtman, R. J., et al. 1984. Alzheimer's disease: Advances in basic research and therapies. Center for Brain Sciences and Metabolism Charitable Trust, P.O. Box 64, Cambridge, Mass.

Yase, Y. 1977. The basic process of amyotrophic lateral sclerosis as reflected in Kii Peninsula and Guam. *Excerpta Medica International Congress,* Series 434, Neurology. 43.

______1980. The role of aluminum in CNS degeneration with interactions of calcium. *Neurotoxicol., 1 (4):* 101-10.

______1987. ALS, + Alzheimer's: Relationship to mineral deficiency and excess aluminum. Personal communication.

Yates, C. M., J. Simpson, D. Russell, and A. Gordon. 1980. Cholinergic enzymes neurofibrillary degeneration produced by aluminum. *Brain Research, 197:* 259-74.

Yokel, R. A. 1982. Hair as an indicator of excessive aluminum exposure. *Clin. Chem., 28 (4):* 662-65.

Yoshimasu, F., Y. Nebayaski, W. Iwata, and K. Sassajima, 1976. Studies on amyotrophic lateral sclerosis by neutron activation and analysis. *Folia Psych. et Neurol., 30:* 49-55.

# Acknowledgments

It is appropriate and important to mention the source of support for the research study I am conducting regarding "Aluminum, Other Metals and Alzheimer's Disease." *Appropriate* because scientific progress is increasingly threatened by institutionalized, highly regimented thinking. Thinking which is controlled by grants more of a political than of an objective, rational nature. *Important* owing to the relative obscure yet medically profound, implications of a gradient shift in thinking evolving as a result of emerging trace metal research in Alzheimer's disease.

Despite numerous appeals, the major foundations refused to fund this epidemiological dietary survey. Luckily, through the foresight and generosity of Eric and Sal Estorick of London, England, the Fund for Ethnic Medicine was able to support this research.

The history of science shows that critical discoveries often hinged on the work of the "private gentleman," those able to pay for their own research, both in time and materials.

> "Without what the English call the 'private gentleman,' the scientific process could not have begun in Greece, and could not have been renewed in Europe. The universities

> played a part, but not a leading part, in the philosophical and scientific thought of this period. Endowed learning is apt to be timid and conservative learning, lacking in initiative and resistant to innovation, unless it has the spur of contact with independent minds."
>
> H.G. Wells *History of the World.*

Today, unless the scientist comes to his study with independent funding, the prospects for conducting truly novel, potentially innovative research are practically nil. Commercial and political interests now dominate the grantmaking process to an almost totalitarian degree of control. Thus, the scientist who sees evidence that aluminum is implicated in Alzheimer's disease faces the resistance both of the medico-pharmaceutical complex and the aluminum industry. Yet the truth which is emerging cannot be suppressed forever. With continued research, perhaps the mounting evidence will be acknowledged. With such acknowledgment, steps will eventually be taken to alert people to the dangers of aluminum and the protective benefits of proper nutritional support.

For those progressive scientists who have shared their initial discoveries with me, I am extremely grateful. For his particular generosity I wish to thank Dr. Armand Lione and the American Pharmaceutical Association.

I am also indebted to Mrs. Sandra Votta for her excellent administrative skills, especially her assistance in organizing the mountain of research papers.

## About the Author

Dr. Michael Savage is a bestselling author, political commentator, activist, and former radio host. The "capstone of his life" was in 2016 when he was inducted into the National Radio Hall of Fame. In 2009, his radio show, *The Savage Nation*, was the second most listened to radio talk show in the United States with over twenty million listeners on four hundred stations.

Savage holds master's degrees in medical botany and medical anthropology, and a PhD in nutritional ethnomedicine from the University of California, Berkeley.

Savage served as the Director of the Alzheimer's Research Institute and is now the host of the top podcast *The Savage Nation* and host of *The Savage Nation* television show on Newsmax TV.

Dr. Savage is the author of over twenty-five books, five of which have been *New York Times* bestsellers and two #1 bestsellers. He is an ardent conservationist, is dedicated to his family, and is a proud patriot of his country.

www.ingramcontent.com/pod-product-compliance
Ingram Content Group UK Ltd.
Pitfield, Milton Keynes, MK11 3LW, UK
UKHW020117290926
15471UKWH00003B/197

9 798895 656501